The Ecology of Care

The Ecology of Care

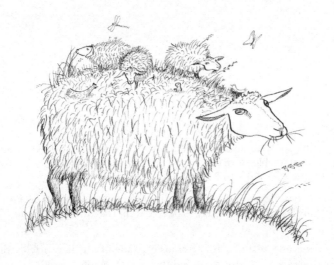

*Medicine, Agriculture, Money, and the Quiet
Power of Human and Microbial Communities*

DIDI PERSHOUSE

MYCELIUM BOOKS

Part of this book originally appeared under the title "Fertile Health: Parallels between Sustainable Agriculture and Sustainable Medicine" on November 20, 2013, on the Post Growth Institute's website.

Excerpts from earlier drafts also appeared in interviews with the author in the *Burlington Free Press* on April 6, 2014, and on the Numen Blog on March 26, 2012.

The chapter on Cuban health care was expanded from an article by the author in *The American Acupuncturist*, Volume XXIII, Winter, 2000.

We are grateful to Bill Peet for inspiring Peter Donovan's sheep illustration on the title page. It was based on Peet's "blue snouted twump" in *No Such Things*. Thanks to Bill Peet Jr. for allowing us to use it.

Mycelium Books
PO Box 277
Thetford Center, VT 05075
(802) 785-2503

This book is typeset in Galliard by Peter Holm at Sterling Hill Productions

Printed in the United States of America

First edition

ISBN-13: 978-0692613030
ISBN-10: 069261303X

To contact the author, to schedule a speaking engagement or workshop, or for questions about book sales, distribution, and educational use, please email: ecologyofcare@gmail.com

More information about the author's work can be found at:
The Center for Sustainable Medicine, www.sustainablemedicine.org
The Soil Carbon Coalition, www.soilcarboncoalition.org

For Henry and Alden,
who cheerfully ate way too many frozen meals
while their mother was writing about health

"If we have no peace, it is because we have
forgotten that we belong to each other."

—Mother Teresa of Calcutta

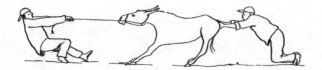

CONTENTS

PREFACE

In the process of writing this book, as I started researching in other disciplines I was faced with the reality that my thinking was not unique. Other systems thinkers were (and still are) coming to similar conclusions in many fields of study. Holmgren's perma-culture principles, for example, are similar to my manifesto points—although I didn't read them till much later. I thought I had coined the term and concepts of what I first called "Ecological Medicine" (and later "Sustainable Medicine"), but I had not: the Bioneers had already published a book of essays under that title.[1] An opening paragraph in Daphne Miller's wonderful book *Farmacology* was a near-exact replica of one in my own, and articles on "Our Inner Ecosystem" started appearing in the *New York Times* and *Scientific American* as I was finishing my first draft of this manuscript—with their authors asking some of the same questions I was.

At times this bothered me, especially as my writing and editing took me so long—as a single parent squeezing writing into the marginal hours of my busy days. But eventually I understood that this co-arising of ideas was simply another reflection of our amazing interconnectedness. It was actually a relief to trade in my sense of uniqueness for a long-desired sense of community, and to trade in my fantasy of becoming a pioneer for the security of moving forward in a pack. The first of many examples of the beauty of community thinking came early on, while I was trying to acquire the domain name "sustainablemedicine.org" for my new website back in 2006.

---

1   The Bioneers and the Science and Environmental Health Network had coined the term "ecological medicine" several years before I used it, and had published an excellent book of transcribed talks on the subject from a Bioneers conference. Joel Kreisberg, a chiropractor, was also using the term "ecologically sustainable medicine" in his work at Teliosis, a nonprofit geared toward "greening" health-care settings and keeping pharmaceuticals out of water supplies.

My "adversary" in this effort, Fiona Robertson, who was holding the domain name for possible future use on the other side of the Atlantic Ocean, turned out to be someone I felt immediately comfortable with (once I stopped bristling at her for owning "my" domain name). We had studied the same obscure medical systems, with many of the same teachers. We were running similar multi-practitioner experimental clinics, were involved in similar social change movements, and were even living similar lives as single women in our forties. Most importantly, we both had a vision of working toward a more sustainable health-care system. We struck up a friendship with a pen pal–like glee that has continued to this day, writing emails and having video chats about everything from government funding for alternative medicine to the ups and downs of romantic relationships. She ended up giving me the domain name for my website as a gift.

The truth is that good ideas, while often credited to one person, are rarely the product of a single individual. Good ideas reflect and work with the patterns and truths that are everywhere and obvious if we only take time to look at them. We see them wherever things are going well, and anyone can access this wisdom. We can tap in to it using collective genius by inviting *everyone* to speak—those who are at the forefront, as well as those who are hidden in the background; those who gravitate toward traditional knowledge, and those who value careful scientific investigation; those who focus on ethical concerns, and those who are known for innovative leaps of the imagination.

There are also patterns and truths that are hard to notice with our usual senses. Sometimes we need to observe with what I think of as our Big Heart, and our Big Mind.

As I listen to others who are bravely tackling the biggest questions, I am reminded over and over again how important it is to cultivate a relationship with the intelligence of the whole. The sanest, bravest, most rational people I know of are those whose work is grounded in a respect for that which enlivens every particle of the universe—whatever they may choose to call it.

As I researched and wrote this book, I had to read through article after article about frightening, upsetting, and urgent situations.
I also experienced a number of crises myself. During those years
it became clearer to me why I need the deep rest, the discipline of
hope, and the uncovering of truth that come from a contemplative
practice. That practice, for me, takes many forms—not all of which
involve closing my eyes, or even sitting still. Listening to the subtle
sounds of a river, staring at every detail of a patch of lichen, singing
out loud as I pick wild raspberries, reading detailed scientific literature deep into the night, and plunging my hands into the warm fur
of my dog while appreciating our interspecies relationship—these
are all examples of my spiritual practice. For me, contemplative life
has two aspects: being *here*, fully engaged and aware, in total gratitude for the chance to participate in this extraordinary world, and
also being quiet enough inside to abide in the wisdom of its ongoing
creation.

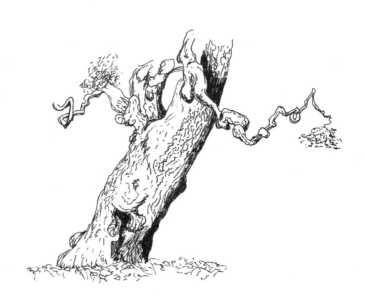

Kitchen Medicine

I live in my clinic these days. I moved in to save money when oil prices spiked and the economy started to collapse, but this cross-pollination of life and work has become a fertile, still-unfolding experiment—with implications I never could have imagined.

In 2008, I was living in a sweet little house on ten acres up in the quiet wooded hills of Thetford Center, Vermont. In the summer chickens roamed around our yard, scratching around the flower beds and eating blueberries. In the winter my two young sons and I painted pictures and played cards in front of the woodstove. The boys could jump off the deck into the snow when the plow pushed it up into six-foot-high piles. Next to the deck was a tremendous old apple tree, where a barred owl often sat keeping me company while I ate breakfast outside.

I had bought the house a few years earlier, when *anyone* could get a mortgage. I had another mortgage and utilities to pay at my clinic, located a few miles down the hill in the village, where I worked as an acupuncturist and rented out office space to friends: a doctor, a massage therapist, and a psychologist. Money was tight as a newly single mother, but credit was easy in those days, so when cash was low I could always put things on a card. After all, interest rates were at zero percent.

There was probably no way I could have seen what was coming: for many years this life had seemed sustainable. Looking back now, I can see how the accumulation of problems that were about to happen in my life were connected with global concerns. At the time, though, it seemed like it was mostly happening to me, and that it was somehow my fault.

It started with a leak in my roof, and then the discovery of termites in the beams. Then two of my colleagues said they could no longer afford to rent office space, which meant our clinic was no longer paying for itself. Patients, many of whom lived more than thirty miles away, started canceling appointments, saying they couldn't afford the gas.

The rates on my old credit card balances suddenly jumped from 0 percent to 11.9 percent, then to 16.9 percent. I got behind in my payments, and late fees piled up. I stopped using credit cards to pay my bills, but I now had some huge debts. Food suddenly seemed more expensive. My electric bill went up, even though I didn't think I was using more, and then my health insurance went up. The phone started ringing with creditors' calls. I was embarrassed, and I was scared. I didn't qualify for public assistance because I "owned" both my house and the clinic. I couldn't sell the house because I owed more on the mortgage than I would be able to sell it for. What had I done wrong that my life was suddenly so unmanageable?

While I was fretting over my bills, the housing market had collapsed, the world economy had gone into a tailspin, and gas prices had hit an all-time high. As things got worse, patients started quietly and embarrassedly confiding in me about their own economic woes.

Several of my patients lost their houses to bank foreclosures, a couple of them ended up homeless, and many others had to move in with family members. The largest employer in our area, a teaching hospital, called the nurses and administrative assistants in to work one day to "reapply for their jobs." A large sign on the wall posted jobs that were still available and jobs that were no longer available, as departments downsized, leaving people angry, and humiliated. Even those who still had seemingly good jobs at the hospital started taking on housecleaning jobs on the side. Men who looked like executives were suddenly bagging groceries at the food coop. It started to dawn on me that perhaps this was not my personal failing, and that perhaps it was time to do things differently.

When I decided to move into my clinic, and shifted to a new way of working that put my rates on a dramatically reduced sliding scale, my patients were delighted. My friends (who didn't realize how much I was struggling financially) were confused. "Why would you want to move out of your wonderful house? Aren't you going to feel weird sleeping in your office?"

I told them it was to make life simpler. "Instead of never being home, now I'll always be home." That was something everyone could relate to.

On this spring morning, before patients arrive, I come down from my bedroom, fry up some eggs and bacon for myself and my now-teenage boys, and send them out the door, piled high with their backpacks, a saxophone, a bass guitar, and baseball gloves.

"I love you!" I yell, over the sound of a truck full of rocks flying by as they drive off to school.

My home/clinic is very much at that fertile edge where the most interesting parts of life happen. I'm on a noisy state highway in a sleepy little town. I'm sandwiched between two garages, but there are well-worn paths behind my house that lead to nearly a thousand acres of forest and meadow owned by the Army Corps of Engineers. Winding its way through this whole messy world of mine is the Ompompanoosuc River—powerful, peaceful, and stunningly beautiful.

The river is cold today—it's April, after all, and this is New England—but I strip down, hop quickly through the otter tracks in the mud, and jump straight in, ducking my head under to feel the current sweeping through my hair. As I emerge, the surface of the water smells beautiful, like the wet moss and ferns that line its banks. I swim quickly across to the rocks, calling my small dog, Phoebe, to join me. She swims like a squirrel, her feathery tail wagging back and forth, making me laugh, and we both circle back around and climb out again. Toweling off, I feel my circulation tingling through my arms and legs, and Phoebe shakes herself down. Now I'm awake and ready to face the day. I walk barefoot back to my clinic, looking for wild edibles and medicinal plants along the way.

As I return from my walk, my assistant, Marisa, arrives wearing a brightly colored wool hat that she will likely have on all day. I've known her since she was seven years old, but now she works for me. It's one of several part-time jobs she juggles as a young adult. She also teaches Chinese, helps a local artist in his printmaking studio, gives tango lessons, and manages the organic farm at the nearby Mountain School. As we clean up the living room before patients arrive, we discuss how the peer-support class we are teaching together went last night, and whether the one person of color in the group is getting annoyed with our awkwardness as we try to welcome her into our rural, overwhelmingly white community.

While my boys are at school, my clinic is open for business. Patients walk through my kitchen on their way in and out of my small consultation office, and share my living room during community acupuncture hours. In the evenings, I teach classes on personal and community resiliency, deep self-care, and peer support for community leaders. I have spent eight years trying to define (and bring into practice) what a truly resilient system of care might look like.

We have developed an extraordinary system of medicine over the past 100 years. We can look inside bodies, map the human genome, restore vision with lasers, transplant hearts, and create new legs that can run at Olympic speeds. For generations, my family has been on the cutting edge of medical and technological innovation, and I know the kind of ego and intense focus that is necessary to explore new and controversial territory. I also know the costs.

Although in many ways science and technology have given us better lives, they also have been used—increasingly—to mine and manipulate the natural resources, biological systems, and communities we rely on for health. That's because for several hundred years both science and religion in Western culture have seen humanity, with its hugely developed frontal lobes, as something quite separate from, and superior to, the rest of nature: more intelligent, more conscious, more spiritual. (Read the introduction to almost any philosophical, spiritual, or scientific book written by a man in the past two centuries and you will likely find a line that lauds humanity's unique capacity for consciousness, intelligence, and/or spirituality.) This perspective has changed the world we are observing, in profound ways. We temporarily lost track of the fact that our existence, our health, and even our consciousness itself is inextricably linked to our environment, and to other organisms, both inside and around us. We are waking up to a world that is almost unrecognizable to our souls and our cells.

Our over-reliance on technology threatens to create new problems as quickly as it solves the old ones. How do we deal with the health challenges of flooding, drought, and wildfires due to climate change; runoff from large industrial farms and factories; and dwindling clean water supplies? How could chronic illness be increasing when scientists know so much more about the human body than they used to? Why are our immune systems becoming compromised or even attacking our own bodies with autoimmune disorders? What do we do about antibiotic-resistant strains of bacteria or "superbugs"? Why are doctors and nurses so burned out?

All these problems stem from our insistence on isolating parts, rather than thinking in terms of our place in the whole. Just as my own personal debt crisis turned out to be related to much larger forces than I could see, our growing "debt" of health and environmental problems is related to larger, more complex issues than we usually assume, and will not be solved by merely fixing individual parts of the system.

We live within a vast interdependent web of relationships, and whatever happens in one part of the system affects the whole. There is no such thing as "human health" apart from the rest of the planet; there is only health. So when I use the word "medicine," I mean something much more profound and far reaching than medical care for humans.

Our current ways of caring—for people, for farm animals, and for land—are based on a limited definition of health and on outdated ideas of "progress," and are mostly directed by corporate interests. Because of this, we have created a situation in which the planet itself has become something like a field hospital, with new species limping in each day in need of help.

The solutions are out there—in fact, they are surprisingly simple—but in order to see them we need to look at larger frames of reference than the ones we've been taught about in school. In particular, we need to pay close attention to places where things are going well.

⚐

When people thrive, you can generally observe that the natural environment around them is also thriving, their relationships are solid, they have abundant, nutrient-dense food to eat and a just society to live in, and they are living in relatively peaceful times.

There are other aspects of health that are harder to see. A person's "microbiome," which comprises the microorganisms residing in and on the body (microorganisms that are constantly repopulated from the landscape around them) turns out to be one of the most important modulators of health, influencing physical and emotional well-being, immunity, and even proper brain development.

Likewise, the microbiology of the soil—which influences local and global water cycles, the climate, and the nutritional quality of our food—is another important modulator of our health, and even of our actual survival. As a health-care provider, I see these two flowing biomes as the essential systems with which, and within which, I work. They are my allies, my teachers, and part of the provenance of my care.

⚹

Living in my workspace turned out to be practical in many ways. I didn't have to pay to heat my home when I was at work, or to heat my clinic when I was at home, or waste all that fuel either. I could pay one electric bill, one oil bill, one phone bill, and have one Internet service. Being able to spread out into the living room and kitchen, I started treating my patients in a group setting so they could split the costs of their appointments, which meant more people could afford to come back and see me. Slowly I started paying down my credit card balances with the money I was saving.

I could chop some onions during a break and keep an eye on supper as I treated patients. My kids could jump on the school bus in the morning, and get off in the afternoon, and I could spend several days at a time without needing to even start the car. After school, I could send my kids down to the post office to mail out a package of medicine, or they could do their homework, and I could do my accounting, side by side. We helped each other figure out problems when we were stuck—and learned a lot about each other's work that way.

If one of my sons had a cold, I didn't have to cancel the whole day's work—I could stash him up in his room and check on him periodically while he slept it off. Snow, sleet, rain, floods? No problem, I was already at work. If patients didn't get here, well, I could catch up on paperwork, or take a nap.

My own kitchen quickly became the heart of the clinic, and food became even more a part of my interaction with patients. I started purposefully cooking soups and stews while working, to help tap into patients' sensory memory of the pleasures of slow food. As people started asking about things they smelled cooking, I started teaching patients more about the connections between diet, health, and soil; about the importance of replenishing their inner ecosystems with nutrient-rich foods brimming with enzymes, natural yeasts, and beneficial bacteria, and how important grass-finished meat, dairy, and eggs are for neurological health.

When patients were unfamiliar with the foods I was describing, I could duck into the kitchen and offer a taste of sauerkraut, kefir, or raw jersey cream, or hand them a recipe for collagen-rich bone broth or eggs benedict, rich in omega-3s. A local foods movement was sprouting up around me, as well, and I started keeping lists of local farms that had the best ingredients. In this way, my patients' lives became more interconnected with my own, in an organic way. Patients often commented that they loved the feeling of entering through my kitchen and being in my home: it tapped in to a sense of care, comfort, and trust that was rarely found in clinical settings. In a sense, I had reinvented the small-town doctor's life, or the village herbalist's.

Meanwhile, my patients started getting healthier, and more interested in taking care of themselves and their families, and a little less dependent on me to help them feel better.

The more I wrote and taught about these ideas, the more I noticed how problems in the areas of health, economics, politics, farming, food, and community are all connected. The solutions are interconnected, as well, as I was discovering in my new life as a health-care provider in the center of a rural village. Things worked better for me and for my patients when my life was scaled down, multipurposed, local, and based on mutual caring and a debt-free microeconomy.

Much of my current life and thinking can be traced back to a piece of paper that I handed out at the Sunfest Expo, in 2007. Sunfest celebrated two themes: Sustainable Living, and Alternative Health. The night before the expo, I was preparing materials to hand out. As I gathered up articles on acupuncture, addictions, herbal medicine, nutrient-dense diets, and more, I was thinking about the expo's two themes, and the connections between ecological sustainability and alternative medicine. I wondered if it were possible to interweave the two ideologies, and if so, what a sustainable model of health care might look like. Who or what would it sustain? Was it just about people, or would it encompass a broader definition of care? Could our current model of medicine fit into it, or was it too dependent on unsustainable technologies? Was all alternative medicine sustainable by default, or would that model need to change, as well?

That night, I began to write down my ideas on what I called "ecological medicine." I came up with a manifesto with defining points that connected human health and environmental health, and the next morning I handed out hundreds of copies. That manifesto grew into a website, which, as my life shifted over the next couple of years, sparked a re-framing and renaming of my clinic from the "Two Rivers Clinic" to "The Center for Sustainable Medicine." For many years I used the term "sustainable medicine," rather than my initial term "ecological medicine," to define my work. But now I think my first take on it was correct: the issue is not so much about sustainability; the issue is about relationships.

The ideas from that original manifesto evolved into a series of talks I presented at hospitals, Transition Town initiatives, conferences, and other gatherings. They wove together with personal conversations—with patients around my kitchen table and with scientists around the world—and finally became this book.

As my understanding has grown, my medical practice has expanded: from treating individuals to treating whole systems. In addition to seeing patients, I now spend time teaching at agricultural conferences and in schools about the interrelationships between healthy soils, shifting weather patterns, economic forces, and human health. I help community leaders create resilient networks of shared support, and I work with farmers and ranchers to restore the quietly powerful living systems that run the underground carbon and water cycles that make life on this planet possible.

The hidden question at the heart of this book is: how do we get close enough to each other so that we can really look out for each other? People are disconnected from each other and nature, and it's obvious in the way we approach health care.

In this book, I will show you how it is all interrelated: care for the land and care for people. I'll show the odd story of what I call the "sterile" industrial model of care, and how we can shift things to a more interconnected, "fertile" way of living and working—from an entire country, to a regional hospital, to the smallest backyard. This approach not only restores our own health, but also restores health to struggling ecosystems both inside and outside the body.

I invite you to contact me, engage with me about these ideas, and let me know if you spot any errors I have made. (A few small details of patients' lives have been changed to protect anonymity.) The benefit of what I call "revolutionary interdependent publishing" (including crowd-source funding, community editing, title brainstorming on social media, and print-on-demand distribution) is that future editions of a book can easily evolve to reflect the larger wisdom of the community that reads it. Welcome to that community.

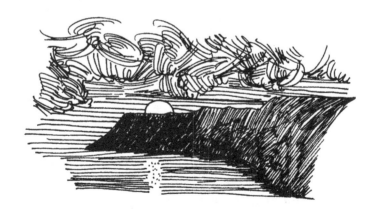

CHAPTER ONE

The Lobotomy of Care

More and more, patients arrive at my doorstep talking about a deep, almost indescribable sense of disconnection. Computer programmers, mothers, bank tellers, factory workers, even artists . . . they all have an uncomfortable sense of separateness. It's as if they had become untethered from the Earth without meaning to, like accidental astronauts: blasted out of the atmosphere by human ingenuity, and suddenly they look around them and want to go home.

"It's as if there is an entire world I've been exiled from. I want to return, but I don't remember it, so how can I describe it?" said a man I sat with yesterday, who yearned to reconnect to some other way of learning that he had lost while being taught to sit still, indoors in elementary school.

Some speak of it as an intense desire to reconnect to nature, not just to go camping or learn the names of plants, but to somehow undo the boundaries of buildings and clothes.

Others feel the pull of a place their family left behind, or a pull to the indigenous culture embodied in the terrain where they now live. They miss those complex bonds that strengthen from generation to generation through shared food, hard work, and wild play.

Some people are so disconnected that a single person, or even a small dog, paying attention to them feels like a miracle.

Disconnection, I am convinced, is at the heart of illness.

After more than twenty years of listening to patients, I've noticed that healing often starts with a desire to reenter the wholes we are born to be part of: landscapes, family and community, and the "is-ness" of life itself.

As a health-care provider—someone whom people come to for both "health" and "care"—I often have the honor of being the first link. As I sit with patients, I listen for the places where I can help them reconnect, whether that means giving them an age-old recipe for bone broth, helping them develop a spiritual practice, or taking them for a walk in the woods with my dog while we talk about widening their support system.

I am constantly aware, however, that this feeling of disconnection that people suffer from is profoundly intertwined with the history and culture of modern medicine and science—and that my own family of origin played a part in that history.

The Brain Surgeon

When I was fifteen, I went to work for my grandfather for a summer, hoping to do what my mother and her two brothers had done. When they were teenagers they assisted him in his surgeries, handing him instruments as he cut into the delicate tissues of the brain and the vulnerable structures of the spine. My grandfather had wanted to be a car mechanic but his father, a lawyer, insisted he take on a profession. So he became, instead, a neurosurgeon at Hartford Hospital and a professor of medicine at Yale. His name was William Beecher Scoville.

Many of the walls in his Frank Lloyd Wright–style house were made of glass from ceiling to floor. They looked out over well-tended gardens and a clear blue swimming pool shaped like a broken rectangle, where my grandfather and his new, young French wife swam naked. Large modern paintings graced the walls, and sleek Scandinavian furniture punctuated the open rooms. As children, my brother and I bicycled up and down the hallways with our aunt and uncle (who were younger than we were). We slid down the staircase on pillows into the huge clean basement, where we played hide-and-seek, snuck gold-wrapped chocolates out of the cupboards, and fell asleep, smelling of chlorine and French perfume, under soft llama-fur throws.

The rules never changed: no gum chewing, and no eating at restaurants. My grandfather's wife, Hélène, served Boston lettuce salad and Dijon vinaigrette every time she roasted a chicken to perfection, and brought my handsome grandfather the same breakfast each morning before work: a boiled egg in an egg cup, a piece of toast, and a small glass of orange juice. He sat and ate it, alone like a king, at the head of the large oval dining room table, while the rest of us sat in the kitchen. The only thing that changed from year to year were the beautiful *au pair* girls; a new one arrived each year from France.

The summer I worked for my grandfather, he left the Rolls Royce in the garage because it was too slow to get to work in, and drove to the hospital each morning in his Mercedes Benz. He was known for driving fast—very fast—and that's what we did on those mornings: 95, 100, 110, even 120 mph. I slid down in the leather seat, closed my eyes, and prayed not to crash as we passed rusty station wagons that looked like the ones my parents drove. But we didn't crash. We threaded our way nimbly through the wealthy suburb onto the highway, past the large corporate headquarters of the insurance agencies whose wealth had built this place, and into the inner city of Hartford.

He gave me a white coat, to differentiate me from the patients, and turned me over to his Scottish secretary, Betty, for training. That summer, I sat in on cases, filed notes, showed patients to their examination rooms, and delivered folders around the hospital, but I never got to help him in his surgeries. That's probably because one particular surgery of his had changed medical history with a flick of a scalpel, and from then on, the world was watching him.

In 1953 (around the time that my mother was handing him his tools), he purposefully removed a portion of the hippocampus from the brain of a young man known as "H.M." in the medical literature, who suffered from nearly constant seizures. The surgery cured the seizures, as my grandfather had hoped it would, but left the patient unable to store new memories. H.M.'s case, followed for

the next fifty-five years by researchers at MIT and McGill, laid the
groundwork for our current understanding of how memory works
in the brain.

⚔

Memory is complex. My own memories have percolated down
through generations, have been infused with stories from friends
and patients, and have been flavored by information from books,
newspapers, and the Internet.

There are other influences on my memory that are larger than
the human stories—or smaller, as the case may be.

When I signal my dog with a tiny movement of my eyes to come
sit with me while I listen to a patient, somewhere in our cells we are
remembering every generation of our human and canine ancestries
that evolved to communicate with each other while working so that
both of us could eat and survive.

When after a long day of work, I jump back into the river one
more time, I bathe in the biochemistry of all the other creatures
that have lived and swum in the river. I walk back home through
a mist of fragrant molecules emitted by the trees that have been
here for hundreds of years before me, and the mushrooms that just
sprang up while I was sleeping the night before. All these molecules
in the air and water interact with my own biochemistry as I move
through the landscape.[1]

When I eat a carrot pulled fresh from the garden, even when I kiss
someone, I am ingesting the modern descendants of ancient strains
of beneficial bacteria and yeasts that have their own cellular memory.
As they populate my inner ecosystem, they influence my development, health, mood, and behavior—and likely my memories as well.[2]

---

1   Li Q, et al., "Forest Bathing Enhances Human Natural Killer Activity and
    Expression of Anti-cancer Proteins," *International Journal of Immunopathology and
    Pharmacology* 20, no. 2 (supplement 2) (2007):3–8.
2   Timothy G. Dinan, et al., "Collective Unconscious: How Gut Microbes Shape
    Human Behavior," *Journal of Psychiatric Research* 63 (2015):1–9.

All of these animals, plants, fungi, yeasts, and bacteria are constantly shifting and changing their chemistry, behavior, and DNA in order to evolve along with each other, and with us, in sickness and in health, like some huge complex vow of love unfolding since the beginning of time.

Lobotomies and Loss of Soul

One of my grandfather's specialties was the lobotomy.

He helped to popularize lobotomies in the 1940s and '50s as a way to relieve symptoms of depression, schizophrenia, and other so-called mental illnesses related to an "excess of emotion."[3] The procedure—so simple that it could be done outside of an operating room—achieved its effect, according to one psychiatrist, by "reducing the complexity of psychic life."[4]

With a quick maneuver, my grandfather sliced the rational frontal lobe free from its web of connections to the deeper, instinctual parts of the brain that we share with other animals. These brain connections, when intact, give us the ability to know instinctively when something is wrong, to respond quickly to dangerous situations, to orient ourselves within a landscape, to pick up subconscious information through our senses, and to discern emotions through subtle shifts in gesture, tone, and smell.

After my grandfather severed the planning and problem-solving "executive" functioning from these more ancient ways of knowing, patients lost something that was hard to pinpoint but easy to notice—and subtly unnerving: there was a general lack of spontaneity, responsiveness, and self-awareness. A colleague of my grandfather's said that the best way to describe what was missing in patients who had had lobotomies was the person's "soul."

3   For a detailed (and somewhat chilling) account of my grandfather's work, see my brother Luke Dittrich's forthcoming book.
4   Maurice Partridge, "Pre-frontal Leucotomy," *British Journal of Surgery* 38, no. 152 (1951):536–37.

His surgeries were just one example of parallel attempts going on all around him to control other unpredictable wildnesses: the insects in our fields, the bacteria in our bodies, the behavior of children, and the tricky emotions of intimate relationships, to name just a few.

Although the practice of lobotomies has ended, the "loss of soul" has not.

With our modern tendency to favor the frontal lobe activities of reductionist, empirical, linear thinking, we have lost our felt sense of our place within the deeper, complex web of life. We have insulated ourselves from that awareness in our everyday lives.

This "soul"—this bridge between reason and instinct—is the essence of what so many of us feel we are missing. If we could find it, it would help us to bring our ancient senses—of orientation, feeling, and relationship—into the conversation as we examine our high-speed modern lives. It would also help us respond to the challenges we currently face with the appropriate mix of urgency and calm, adaptation and resiliency.

I suspect that while most of us have never suffered a lobotomy, we have been impacted by the same forces that made my grandfather and his colleagues decide, over and over again, that this severing of reason from response was the only recourse: a need to soothe anxieties, reduce variables, and control the wild unpredictability of life and emotions in an era of rapid change.

The Dove Laboratory

On a winter day in 1984, as my grandfather exited the highway, another car slammed into his, killing him instantly. He was seventy-eight years old, still working full time as a brain surgeon. I was in college.

It was the end of an era in our family's life. There would be no more wild card games around the huge table, no more riding bicycles down the halls, no more caviar or Rolls Royces. No one else could really take his larger-than-life place, and so we simply stopped gathering.

But on some other level, he was truly indestructible. Lying in my dorm room thinking about him after his death, I felt a strange sensation, almost as if something from his life was being poured into mine. I wasn't sure I wanted it, but he wasn't that kind of giver.

The sensation reminded me of how I'd felt after a short conversation with him a few months before. He had pulled me aside in private at a holiday gathering, and asked me about my life. It was rare to get private attention from him, but perhaps he had already heard the news that the rest of us didn't find out about until after the car accident: that he had a rare form of cancer. He pulled out a small box and opened it to reveal a pair of lavish gold and amethyst earrings shaped like upside-down question marks.

"Here," he said, putting the box in my hands somewhat awkwardly. "This is just between you and me. You have a good mind and I admire what you are doing—studying Chinese and Russian. These were given to me by a patient in South America. I think you are the only one in the family who can handle them."

The sense in that earlier moment was the same kind of feeling I felt now in my dorm room after his death: it was such a surprise to be given anything by him that I felt compelled to accept. As I pondered my odd inheritance, I wasn't sure I wanted either of them—the earrings or his inspiration—but I was determined to make them my own.

⚔

A few months after my grandfather died, I applied for a work-study job in the neuropsychology laboratory at my college. My job was to take care of hundreds of ring-necked doves, each living an isolated life in its own little metal cage in upper Manhattan. One day, as I was cleaning out cages, the woman who ran the psychology lab invited me to see what the birds were used for.

She had a dove clamped into a small metal box, looking quite confused. The top of the bird's skull had been removed, without anesthesia, exposing the miniature brain inside. She paused— holding her tiny tools in midair, before she dove in to remove some part of the brain—to explain how this surgery would allow her to observe changes in the bird's memory and behavior. She must have seen me wince, because she assured me in a cool voice that it didn't hurt—it couldn't possibly—because birds don't have the same relationship to pain as humans do.

It was hard to get the image out of my mind later, as I held the other doves, cleaned their cages, and gave them seeds and water.

Here is what I observed: every day I poured a colorful mix of twenty different seed varieties into their feeding boxes, yet each dove had one or two types of seeds that he or she disliked. So, over time, each clear plastic box filled up with a different kind of rejected seed, making a patchwork of natural colors that was visually appealing to me. It was the only variation in the otherwise stark rows of identical cages.

This got me thinking about medical research itself. These doves were considered, for experimental purposes, to be a large group of identical units. But they weren't. Each dove was different, with individual tastes and preferences, and although the researchers were intending to feed the birds all the same food, in fact they had different diets, by choice.

They were also living entirely non-dove-like lives. Totally absent were such stimuli as flight and navigation, sunlight and moonlight, treetop and meadow, probably leaving those parts of their brains woefully undeveloped. Also absent was any experience of relationship, courtship, or flock behavior. In this entirely artificial and human-made environment, how could the scientists fully understand the changes they were observing?

I shared my thoughts with the woman who ran the lab, but she seemed to have little interest in my perspective. She was working in the reductionist, empirical model of science, trying to understand things by separating them from their natural environment and taking them apart, piece by piece.

I, on the other hand, was thinking about whether I could get away with opening all the cages and windows and letting the doves reunite with the earth- and sky-filled world to which they belonged.

The Radioactive Family

Although I was unaware of it at the time, the animal laboratory I worked in was an offshoot of my *great*-grandfather's animal laboratory, which he ran when he was director of the Crocker Institute of Cancer Research and director of the pathology laboratory at Saint Luke's Hospital from 1910 to 1948.[5] He was my father's grandfather, Dr. Francis Carter Wood, known to his family as Poppy. On weekends he experimented with the latest technology—photography—taking pictures of his children sitting in prams with their large bonnets and bows in Central Park, or posing on their summer porch in Claremont, New Hampshire, with their mother in her high-necked Victorian dresses.

The rest of the week he experimented with radiation—X-rays and radium—to diagnose and treat cancer. He and Marie Curie corresponded across the Atlantic, and he helped raise money from women in the United States so Curie could buy radioactive materials for her work. He also pioneered the use of laboratory animals for cancer research. As a professor at Columbia, his daughters got free tuition at Barnard, the women's college across the street. I followed my grandmother's footsteps to Barnard, and my great-grandfather's lab full of rabbits and rats became my lab full of ring-necked doves.

His legacy was passed down in an unusual way: he experimented on a number of our family members, "successfully" treating my

5   Wilhemina F. Dunning, "Francis Carter Wood, 1869–1951," *American Journal of Cancer* 11 (1951):296.

grandmother's acne, my father's sore throats, and my great-uncle's warts—with radiation.

Radiation was all the rage in those days. At the World's Fair, people tried out sitting in radioactive baths as amusement, to feel the fizzy sensations. Shoe salesmen had X-ray machines where you could see the bones of your feet when you stood on them and wiggled your toes. But over the course of my great-grandfather's lifetime, it became more and more obvious that radiation—while amusing to play with, and therapeutic in some ways—had problematic results. Many of my relatives suffered side effects from his treatments: thyroid problems, skin cancer, and other afflictions related to the radiation that had changed the DNA of their cells.

Near the end of the Second World War, scientists from the Manhattan Project called my great-grandfather Wood into a meeting to discuss the likely aftereffects of dropping an atomic bomb on Japan. My family still remembers him coming home that day, shaking his head in disbelief and discouragement at how his research on radioactivity and cancer—intended to help humanity—was being used for something so destructive.

This was not unusual for the era; science and technology crisscrossed the boundaries of medical, agricultural, and military lines. Rat poisons became blood thinners, pesticides became poison gas, agricultural herbicides were used as defoliants to uncover enemies in military operations, and chemicals left over from the manufacture of bombs became fertilizers for farms and ingredients in toothpaste.

I never was brave enough to let the doves out while I worked in the lab. Yet that unfulfilled urge for a change has worked within me over the years, making me constantly question whether there is something missing in the world of medicine, some other way of knowing that sees individual health as inseparable from the inner and outer landscapes in which we were born. Something the person taking care of the doves could contribute to the fields of medicine, science, and memory.

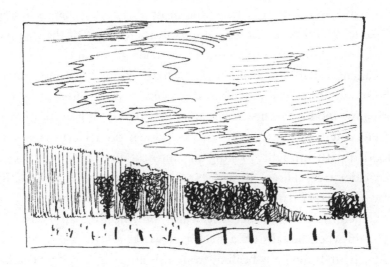

A Day at the Clinic: The Farmer and the Acupuncturist

Phoebe barks. My first patient, Ted, is at the door.

He drops off some butter and milk in my refrigerator as he comes in, gives me a hug, and asks me where he should put the potatoes, eggs, and beef he has brought, as well. My assistant, Marisa, and I smile at each other—it's a rare treat to see Ted, and we look forward to the food he brings. He's one of those farmers who focuses on quality: breeding heirloom cows from generations of healthy stock, all raised outdoors on pure pasture. I've treated his family for years.

In a rural town like Thetford, with a population of 2,700, relationships are—by nature—multilayered and complex.

One patient might be a neighbor who plows my driveway and lends me tools. Another might be the owner of my favorite dance hall *and* the person who carved my salad bowl. Yet another is my best friend's sister-in-law, the person I buy gas from, *and* my house cleaner.

Many relationships have shifted and deepened since I first opened my acupuncture practice here more than twenty years ago. Strict, socially "sterile" boundaries between patient and provider are impossible in my practice here, and most of the time that's the way I like it. It allows me to see patients in the context of their actual lives, and allows them to see me in the context of mine.

Patients call me on my home phone to set up appointments, shovel the snow off my walkway when they see I'm super-busy, and often bring me food from their farms and kitchens. Ted is no exception.

He enters the next room and lies down on a treatment table flooded with sunlight, looking out into the understory of a large box-elder tree. Three chickadees, a blue jay, and two doves shift places in a jazzy dance between branches and the ground.

Generally, Ted is in excellent health, only needing an occasional tune-up when he falls off a tractor or works a little too hard. But today he tells me he is healing from a shoulder injury, he has a bit of a fever, and he is trying to get off the sleeping pills he has been using every once in a while since his wife died. As he speaks, I listen not just for information about his symptoms, but also to the tone of his voice, which sounds tired but not exhausted. As he answers me, I notice the lack of sparkle in his eyes.

I feel his pulse, which helps me to pinpoint which parts of his body are holding tension or have poor circulation; whether he is fighting off an acute or chronic infection; as well as how his heart is working. I look at his tongue for odd variations in color, coating, cracks, or shape, which would alert me to deeper changes in his gut flora and interior organs—the beginnings of more serious problems.

My diagnostic tools are not machines; they are my own senses. As I move around his body, I can smell that he is basically healthy, just as I can smell when other patients are not. I can feel from the skin on his forearm and ankles that he is getting enough fats from the grass-fed cream and butter he eats to keep it supple and warm, and from the tone of his muscles that he is getting enough protein. From the way his skin bounces back when pressed, I can feel that his lymphatic system is in good order, which means that he is getting enough exercise and drinking enough fluid.

He starts to relax as he feels my warm hands on his wrists, arms, and feet, and his breathing settles down.

I learned to touch and feel my patients from the blind acupuncturists I studied with in Japan,[6] and have combined it with my own knowledge of biomedicine, nutrition, and many years of practice. But the importance of the *way* I touch patients is deeper than diagnostics. Modern life deprives us of touch at every turn: from the moment we are put into a crib, to the years we spend alone in nursing homes. One of my blind teachers, Toshio Yanagishita, said to me, "As soon as you touch the patient, the treatment has begun."

I slip a few hair-thin needles into Ted's wrists, ankles, and ear, and within minutes he is sound asleep.

Often he comes for a private visit, so we have more time for talking, but today is one of my community days. Every 15–20 minutes— while Ted's treatment continues—I start a treatment with a new patient, on my couch, in an armchair, on another treatment table. Over the next hour, a stressed-out real estate broker seeking relief from migraines, a young tattooed woman recovering from a heroin addiction, and a retired police officer dealing with nightmares all share this treatment room. As Ted drifts in and out of a nap, he hears the hum of my conversation with each person as they arrive: one person makes me laugh, with his thick Boston accent, full of outrageously funny curses; another one quietly whispers and briefly breaks into tears. The stories blend into each other, as I throw in my own anecdotes. Long stretches of quiet fill in most of the space, and there is a mammalian comfort in the air. We are bodies, hearts, and minds: working, resting, snoring. A back exposed here, a thigh there, a shoulder over there.

The costs are minimal because the technology is simple, the relationships are complex, and the resources are shared.

---

6   Acupuncture is the traditional profession for the blind in Japan.

✄

Ted's farm, like my practice, has a certain relaxed efficiency, based
on complexity. In spring, summer, and fall, his cows spend their
days grazing in pastures along the Connecticut River. In the coldest
months of winter, the cows eat hay—the same food—but cut and
dried from Ted's own fields. As the cattle move their heavy bodies
through the landscape, their hooves press seeds into the ground
and their manure restores fertile microorganisms to the topsoil.

The soil itself is a complex carbon-based food web in which a
multistoried community of plants use water, CO_2, and sunlight to
create sugars that ultimately feed all the life on the farm, including
the mycorrhizal fungi which extend the plants' root systems and
make water and minerals available to the plants. The fungi, related
closely to animals, act as an intelligent filter that can exclude toxins
while searching out and transporting nutrients back to the plants
that need them. Other fungi and bacteria break down dead and
decaying plant material, turning it into fertile soil humus. Larger
microorganisms—nematodes and microarthropods—feed on the
smaller microorganisms. Insects, earthworms, and small burrow-
ing animals aerate the soil and attract birds and larger animals.
Pollinators thrive on the multitude of flowering plants, and keep
the cycle moving. Biodiversity rules.

There is a circle of care in Ted's home life, as well: his parents
live with him, so he can help them as they age, while they help him
with his farm, and with his son. Almost everything around him is
multipurposed. The manure from Ted's milking barn is spread on
his garden, fertilizing the plants. Chickens eat the surplus milk that
has gone sour, as well as scraps from the kitchen. The well-fed hens,
in turn, provide the community with eggs.

Ted's circular farming practices create nutrient-dense foods that
prevent and treat exactly the sorts of modern health problems I see
in my practice: heart disease, allergies, diabetes, attention disorders,
infertility, gut problems, depression, and Alzheimer's.

The pasture-raised meat, eggs, and dairy products here are high in omega-3 fatty acids and other healthy fats that stabilize blood sugar, improve nerve and brain function, balance hormone levels, and reduce inflammation. The vegetables and fruits Ted grows for his family and friends are packed with vitamins, minerals, and other micronutrients precisely because the soil on his farm is full of the microbial life that is necessary to extract minerals from the sand, silt, and clay, and—with the help of sunlight and water—turn them into nourishing food for larger life forms. Ted's mother lacto-ferments some of the vegetables and dairy products to create probiotic foods that restore the beneficial bacteria necessary for healthy immune systems and biochemical balance in the body's inner ecosystem.

Food is medicine we take three times a day. His farm is a veritable pharmacy.

✄

When Ted's treatment is over, Marisa and I offer him a bowl of the chowder we are having for lunch, made with his potatoes, onions, and heavy cream, and we sit together talking during a lull in the afternoon schedule. As he leaves, he chats for a moment on the porch with a friend who is arriving. I duck out and ask him if he can give another patient a ride up the hill.

There is something very satisfying about the fact that the food from Ted's farm gives me energy to do my work, and my work gives him energy to provide me with food.

Our work is part of a cycle—an enormous fertile, creative cycle—that has been going on for billions of years.

The power goes out often in Vermont: windstorms and ice storms knock trees from our heavily wooded landscape onto power lines. But his farm and my clinic are barely affected. If a more serious disaster happened and deliveries of supplies were interrupted, we would still have many time-tested tools to work with, and we would still be able to provide our communities with two of life's necessities: food and care. When practiced in "fertile" ways, both are life-sustaining forms of nourishment.

Our work is integrated into our particular landscape, but fertile models of care can happen anywhere: in cities, large hospitals, and even rooftop gardens. It's a shift in both diagnosis and treatment: a shift from working on parts toward working within wholes.

How did we get so far away from integrated models of care?

Dirty Cows and Whiskey Sludge: The Germ Theory of Disease

"I beseech you to take interest in these sacred domains so expressively called laboratories. Ask that there be more and that they be adorned, for these are the temples of the future, wealth, and well-being. It is here that humanity will grow, strengthen, and improve."

—**Louis Pasteur, microbiologist and chemist, in 1878**[7]

Cows, like Ted's, did not adapt well to the Industrial Revolution.

As industrialized cities became larger, more polluted, and more crowded in the 1800s, food needed to be transported longer distances, and spoilage became an issue. Fresh milk was particularly difficult to procure, because it spoiled so easily in warm weather, and—as the "commons," or common grazing areas, in cities were turned over to development—there was little or no space for cows to graze within city limits. In the early 1800s, entrepreneurs in New York City came up with a brilliant and profitable solution: keep the cows indoors next to the whiskey distilleries and feed them the sludge left over from whiskey production.[8]

Suddenly fresh milk from these cows was available to city resi-

7   Celerino Abad-Zapatero, *Crystals and Life: A Personal Journey* (La Jolla: International University Line, 2002), 139.
8   Ron Schmid, *The Untold Story of Milk: Green Pastures, Contented Cows and Raw Dairy Foods* (Washington, DC: New Trends Publishing, 2003).

dents, and it sold like crazy.[9] Unfortunately, cows can't be kept indoors and fed whiskey sludge without developing serious illnesses; they typically survived only a year under these conditions.[10] Bacteria from these sick cows ended up in the milk supply, and without refrigeration they multiplied easily, along with other bacteria, such as *E. coli* and *Salmonella,* related to the filthy conditions of the dairies. "Slop dairy" from distilleries became a serious vector for disease in cities in the United States and Europe. Infant mortality in cities rose sharply after the distillery dairies began to sell the infected milk—climbing from 32 percent to 50 percent in just twenty-five years in New York City.[11,12]

This stubborn insistence of cows—to live in healthy surroundings, *or else*—was one of several factors that would ultimately drive science, agriculture, and medicine into the modern era: an era that valued a new, sterile paradigm, replacing the fertile paradigm that had defined humans' relationship to life up to that point.

During the 1850s, while distillery dairies were still thriving, Louis Pasteur, a French microbiologist and chemist, lost three of his five children (at ages two, nine, and twelve) to typhoid fever, a food-borne illness caused by *Salmonella* bacteria. Pasteur's research—already focused on the role of microorganisms in the process of fermentation—soon proved that heating foods, like milk, to high temperatures, and then sealing them (now called pasteurization) inhibited the growth of bacteria.[13] By showing that microorganisms

9   In 1852, three-quarters of the money spent on milk by New York City's 700,000 residents was spent on "slop milk" from distilleries. Ralph Selitzer, *The Dairy Industry in America* (New York: Books for Industry, 1976), 123.
10 Robert M. Hartley, *An Historical, Scientific and Practical Essay on Milk as an Article of Human Sustenance* (New York: J. Leavitt, 1842), 67–68.
11 Ron Schmid, *The Untold Story of Milk: Green Pastures, Contented Cows and Raw Dairy Foods* (Washington, DC: New Trends Publishing, 2003).
12 Feedlots for beef cattle were developed during this same period, starting on the south side of Chicago. Feedlots were made possible by the developments of the Industrial Revolution: trains to transport cattle, and tractors which created a surplus of corn and other grains for feed. Philip D. Hubbs, "The Origins and Consequences of the American Feedlot" (Thesis, Baylor University, History Department, 2010).
13 We have since learned that pasteurized milk—and many other industrially produced food products, such as deli meats, spinach, and eggs—can still be responsible for

were the cause of food spoilage and food-borne illnesses, Pasteur solidified the germ theory of disease. This ultimately created a sea change in medicine—as well as in human life. People, animals, and food started to be seen as potentially dirty and unsafe, because they could carry germs.

Laboratories and scientists, on the other hand, were clean.

Before the germ theory of disease took hold, doctors performing surgery were almost absurdly unconcerned with cleanliness. Surgeons' hands, rarely washed, were placed directly into the patient's wounds. Onlookers were encouraged to "take a feel" for educational purposes. Surgeons wore clothing covered in blood, as proof of their "popularity."[14] (In fact, surgeons garnered little respect in those days, and were seen only as a last resort for desperate patients.) Surgical instruments were crudely wiped, placed back into their velvet carriers, and reused, some having been sharpened on the sole of the surgeon's boot. The floors of surgical wards were covered with human feces, urine, blood, and pus, and the hospital walls displayed a collage of phlegm and other body fluids. Consequently, infection was a major cause of death in the early 1800s, with 80 percent of operations plagued by "hospital gangrene" and a nearly 50 percent mortality rate.[15]

When Ignaz Semmelweis suggested (based on his observation of midwives) in 1847 that handwashing with a chlorine solution might be a useful addition to surgical practice, he was ruthlessly mocked by his peers; he ended up dying in an insane asylum.

Pasteur and his contemporaries changed all that. Joseph Lister

serious bacterial illnesses. Between 1980 and 2005, forty-one outbreaks, attributing 19,531 illnesses to the consumption of pasteurized milk and milk products, were reported to the CDC. The largest outbreak of salmonella in US history was from pasteurized milk from an industrial farm. C. A. Ryan, et al., "Massive Outbreak of Antimicrobial-Resistant Salmonellosis Traced to Pasteurized Milk," *JAMA* 258, no. 22 (1987):3269–74.

14 Jason T. Miller, et al., "The History of Infection Control and its Contributions to the Success and Development of Brain Tumor Operations," *Neurosurgical Focus* 18, no. 4 (2005):1–5.

15 Ibid.

started using carbolic acid to sterilize tools and clean wounds in 1867. Lister wrote about his method in the *Lancet*, and included suggestions to stop using porous materials in the handles of surgical tools, thus bringing surgery to a new level of safety. Handwashing finally became standard surgical procedure. As the death and infection rates from surgeries plummeted, surgeons were able to confidently explore and repair the human body, and surgery developed into a highly specialized and respected medical profession.

The creation of a sterile field, which was so essential for surgery, became the hallmark of all of modern medicine. Soon all doctors and scientists, not just surgeons, donned white coats as a symbol of the new era: a signal to the public of a new form of medicine, one that would not allow microorganisms to interfere with human life.

Magic Bullets: Modern Medicine as a Gateway to Reliance on Technology.

The horrendous conditions of World Wars I and II and the spread of disease through the newly industrialized world greatly increased the pressure to develop an antibiotic drug to treat the wave of illnesses that were cropping up. In 1939, before World War II ended, a powerful and wide-acting form of penicillin was finally manufactured for commercial use.[16] Once available, it easily cured many infections that had previously been untreatable, such as syphilis, pneumonia, and wound infections.

The dirty industrial era shifted toward the clean technological era, with medicine at the forefront, and the race was on. If we

---

16 The widespread use and production of antibiotics began in 1939, when microbiologist René Dubos isolated the compounds gramicidin and tyrocidine from the soil bacteria *Bacillus brevis*. These became the first commercially produced antibiotics. Dubos's discovery also revived scientists' interest in researching penicillin—which had been used for centuries by herbalists. Dubos, interestingly, was also an environmentalist. He coined the phrase "Think Globally, Act Locally" and warned about the danger of bacteria developing resistance to antibiotics as early as 1942. See Andrew C. Revkin "A 'Despairing Optimist' Considered Anew," *New York Times*, June 6, 2011.

could eliminate all germs, stop pain with anesthesia, and surgically repair any mechanical problems, we could essentially put an end to disease.

Penicillin became the gateway drug for generations of other drugs, creating the hope that scientists working in laboratories would eventually find a "magic bullet" for each and every illness, one that could cure, like penicillin did, in a matter of days or weeks. All we needed to do was aim the right bullet at each invader, and health would be restored.

Medicine, agriculture, and politics all used similar metaphors. War was increasingly seen as a kind of "medicine" to rid society of unwanted elements, and medicine and agriculture were increasingly seen as a kind of "war"—against bacteria, viruses, and insects. It seemed for a while that anything in society that was unwanted could easily be eradicated: garden pests, tooth decay, blood clots, "defective" populations, even "mental illness."

We have left some of these ideas firmly in the past, yet the underlying mind-set—that technology and science will solve all our problems as we enter the future—persists. As we speak, scientists just down the street from where I grew up are perfecting deep-brain stimulation devices for people with depression, and genetically engineered tomatoes in which to grow vaccines.

In the same way that the successes of antibiotics created huge expectations for new drug development, modern medicine as a whole became the "gateway drug" for our ever-increasing reliance on technology. The early successes of modern medicine satisfied such a deep survival need in humans that many people broadly assumed that *anything* innovative, "scientific," or technological was somehow not only an improvement, but also necessary for our evolution, if not our very survival.

Pasteur was looking through a small frame. His model, developed in the unhealthy depths of the Industrial Revolution, had a targeted goal to solve a specific problem. The medical and agricultural researchers who followed his lead aimed to eliminate "problems" wholesale, rather than understanding the complex role that microorganisms, "weeds," and insects play in the larger, fertile world of biological diversity: the world of meadows, sunshine, and clear, cool rivers that the sickly, whiskey-sludge cows were yearning for.

From hand sanitizers to Lysol, the illusion of sterility still permeates our daily lives, dangling an unfulfilled promise of health. While there have been some definite short-term gains for humans, there have been some enormous long-term losses for everything else.

I respect medical innovation and all that it has added to our lives; however, in my own lifetime I see that the shift toward a more "sterile" industrialized model of care—isolating parts, killing off whatever is not wanted, and relying purely on high-tech solutions to life's problems—can sometimes be a dangerous ride. Like my own family's history, it's a freewheeling, fast-moving experiment with unknowable consequences.

The "Sterile" Model of Care

"People are fed by the food industry, which pays no attention to health, and are treated by the health industry, which pays no attention to food."
—Wendell Berry

At large industrial farms, animals are fed a diet of corn and soybeans, genetically engineered to withstand heavy doses of agricultural chemicals—typically sold by the same company that makes the genetically altered seeds. The application of pesticides, herbicides, and fungicides, along with the tilling of the soil, create a "clean slate." These chemicals work hard to kill off almost everything other than the crop itself, including the deep-rooted native plants, mycorrhizal fungi, pollinators, earthworms, and other microorganisms that create the living structure of the soil.[17] With less biodiversity above ground, there are fewer microorganisms below ground to break down the naturally occurring minerals in the soil and make them available to plants, so expensive chemical fertilizers must be added. The soil, in turn, becomes a relatively inert substance used to prop up plants, rather than a living ecosystem.[18]

Once its living structure collapses, the soil loses its natural carbon-rich, moisture-holding capacity, so it also needs irrigation. The irrigation is really no better than the rain: it runs off the dirt easily, carrying silt and chemicals downstream and creating "dead zones" in rivers, lakes, and oceans. The practice of chemical agriculture also leaves farmers hugely dependent on large corporations that set the prices for genetically engineered seeds and the ever-increasing doses of chemicals that go with them.

Without the mycorrhizal fungi as intelligent living filters, plants lose the ability to measure their intake of—and differentiate between—toxins and nutrients. Plants growing in heavily treated soils take up lead, arsenic, and other excessive minerals, and cannot solubilize the ones they need, like selenium and iron. They can become both toxic and nutrient-deficient as foods, resulting in unhealthy plants, animals, and people.[19]

The fat tissues in animals absorb the chemicals in their feed—cancer-causing dioxins, in particular—which are then passed along to those who eat factory-farmed animal products.[20] Confined animals eating industrial foods are more likely to become sick, so their feed is supplemented with a constant stream of antibiotics (both intentionally and incidentally with antimicrobial Glyphosate residues[21]) to prevent

17 "Glyphosate Interactions with Physiology, Nutrition, and Diseases of Plants: Threat to Agricultural Sustainability?" *European Journal of Agronomy* 31 (2009):111–13.
18 Elaine Ingham, Lecture, Northeast Organic Farming Association Summer Conference, 2014.
19 Walter Jehne, lecture and private interviews following the "Restoring Water Cycles to Reverse Global Warming" conference, Tufts University, October 2015.
20 http://www.who.int/mediacentre/factsheets/fs225/en/.
21 Monsanto patented Glyphosate (Roundup®) as a broad-spectrum antimicrobial, as well as an herbicide.

infection and make them grow faster. The scientific community agrees that antibiotic use in beef, chicken, and pork farming contributes directly to the number of antibiotic-resistant infections that now plague hospitals, like the one where I gave birth to my two sons.[22,23]

⚔

You'd never guess there was a problem with antibiotic-resistant infections at this hospital, because the large modern hallways are gleaming, the ceilings are high and airy, and light pours in through huge sparkling-clean windows. Someone plays a grand piano as you walk into the spacious entrance hall. Everything about the place speaks of professionalism, privacy, sterility, and wealth. It's a bit like entering a very exclusive hotel.

Patients are asked to stand back from the desk while waiting in line with the receptionist so no one overhears anyone else's information. If a patient is admitted to the hospital and her best friend is in the room next door, nurses are not allowed to tell either of them that the other one is there.

It's not just the patients that are sequestered from the complexity of their natural communities. The medicines that doctors prescribe at this hospital are also far removed from the complex herbs, ecosystems, and cultural traditions that inspired their development and use. Instead, they are simple chemical compounds: often petroleum-based replicas of a single plant alkaloid, without variation, packaged in plastic with computer-generated instructions, handed out by pharmacists in white jackets, and billed to an insurance company.

---

22 John Conley, "Antimicrobial Resistance: Revisiting the 'Tragedy of the Commons,'" *Bulletin of the World Health Organization* 88, no. 11 (2010) 797–876, http://www.who.int/bulletin/volumes/88/11/10-031110/en/index.html.

23 "III. The Environmental Impact of Imprudent Antimicrobial Use in Animals," Antimicrobial Resistance Learning Site, http://amrls.cvm.msu.edu/veterinary-public-health-module/iii.-the-environmental-impact-of-imprudent-antimicrobial-use-in-animals/iii.-the-environmental-impact-of-imprudent-antimicrobial-use-in-animals.

False Positives

Over-reliance on machine- and laboratory-based diagnostics has also created new issues in medicine. The "over-detection," or false positives, in high-tech medical testing leads to dangerous exploratory surgeries, further testing with radioactive dyes, and even unnecessary treatment—all of which carry new risks. Some of these risks fall on patients who were perfectly healthy in the first place. Nearly 10 percent of women screened by a blood test for ovarian cancer, for example, have falsely positive results, and of these, one-third have unnecessary surgery, usually to remove one or both ovaries. At least 15 percent of those have at least one serious complication, such as blood clots, infections, or injuries to other organs. Yet due to a variety of pressures, one-third of doctors still recommend this screening, even though patients who are screened have no higher chance of survival than those who are not. Put another way: to find one case of ovarian cancer via a blood test, nineteen healthy women have to undergo surgery.*

---

*   Denise Grady, "Ovarian Cancer Screenings Are Not Effective, Panel Says," *New York Times*, September 10, 2012.

Because the drugs in mainstream medicine are so potent, patients have a small but real chance of dying from the drugs the hospital prescribes for them, and an even higher chance of developing serious complications.[24,25] The occasional medicines that patients truly need are not the problem. It is the nonessential ones that have flooded the system—pushed by marketers from pharmaceutical

---

24   J. Lazarou, et al., "Incidence of Adverse Drug Reactions in Hospitalized Patients: A Meta-Analysis of Prospective Studies," JAMA 279, no. 15 (1998):1200–1205.
25   "To Err is Human: Building a Safer Health System," Institute of Medicine, Report, 1999.

companies at huge financial cost to the consumer—which create minuscule benefits and substantial risks. In fact, according to one study, iatrogenic issues—things like medical and pharmaceutical errors and hospital-acquired infections—are the number one cause of death in the United States.[26]

Although the cancer-causing dioxins from medical incinerators are mostly filtered out these days, this sparkling clean hospital —like *all* hospitals—has a large stream of waste. This includes radioactive waste from CT scans and other diagnostic techniques, drug waste, and tons of disposable plastic tubes, bags, syringes, and instruments—about one ton for every 100 patients. According to the US Department of Energy website, hospitals use 836 trillion BTUs of energy annually, have more than 2.5 times the energy usage and CO_2 emissions of commercial office buildings, and produce more than 30 pounds of CO_2 emissions per square foot.[27]

There is nothing surprising about any of this; in fact, this hospital is considered ahead of the curve, both in standards of medical care and environmentally sound practices. It's just that the kind of high-tech care they provide uses a lot of nonrenewable resources and therefore takes a toll on the environment, by its very nature.

The Creation of a Medical Monoculture

There is a reason that the US health-care system insists on using high-tech, high-profit solutions to human illnesses, rather than focusing on prevention, community health, and other more ecological, systems-based approaches (even though these have been shown to be more efficient and low cost). Our current medical system was purposefully developed in a socially sterile "test tube" of an

26 Gary Null, et al., "Death by Medicine," *Life Extension Magazine*, March 2004.
27 "Department of Energy Announces the Launch of the Hospital Energy Alliance to Increase Energy Efficiency in the Healthcare Sector," US Department of Energy.

environment, genetically engineered to highlight certain traits and eliminate others.

In the late 1800s, there was still as much diversity in the medical field as there is in the meadow behind my clinic. Medical providers included many types of doctors: eclectics, homeopaths, osteopaths, chiropractors, naturopaths, surgeons, and "regular" doctors, just to name a few, all on relatively equal footing. In addition, there were local herbalists, midwives, and parish nurses. Most of these practitioners viewed health and the human body in a holistic, systems-based way.[28,29] Some hospitals and medical schools employed a variety of practitioners all practicing under the same roof, while specialized schools and hospitals nourished particular niches of knowledge. (At the turn of the century, for example, there were more than twenty homeopathic medical schools in the US, and more than 100 homeopathic hospitals.[30])

Only a portion of doctors were practicing the kind of medicine that looks at things through dissection and microscopes, rather than taking a larger, ecological view. But there was a parallel shift going on in the politics and economics of medicine that turned the small but important idea of *surgical* sterility into a worldwide campaign to eliminate anything that threatened the white coats of MDs.

Two streams—the germ theory of disease, and a struggle for economic power and control—converged into a tidal wave that crashed over the medical landscape and swept all other views of health out to sea. It came to a head when a group of well-meaning but competitive doctors performed a radical surgery—with a hatchet, not a scalpel—on the US health-care system in its youthful years. It removed a portion of our collective memory, and altered the future of medicine in the United States.

28 Paul Starr, *The Social Transformation of American Medicine* (New York: Basic, 1982).

29 Barbara Griggs, *Green Pharmacy: The History and Evolution of Western Herbal Medicine* (Rochester, Vermont: Healing Arts Press, 1997).

30 Dana Ullman, *Homeopathy: Medicine for the 21st Century* (Berkeley: North Atlantic Books, 1987).

The homeopaths, who had been very popular with the general public because of the safety and low cost of their medicines, had just started a national association from which they launched attacks on the "regular" doctors and their "heroic" methods—things like bloodletting, dangerous surgeries, and large doses of mercury and laxatives to treat nearly everything. In 1847, the "regular" doctors, in response, started the American Medical Association (AMA), creating a board to "analyze quack remedies and enlighten the public in regard to the nature and danger of such remedies."[31] Homeopaths, naturopaths, botanical practitioners, and other ecologically minded "quacks" were not allowed into the AMA. Regular doctors could lose their license even for consulting with them.[32]

The movement to consolidate professionals in order to have more power reflected a larger trend that was sweeping the nation: the corporation. Business models of efficiency, run by "experts," were replacing personal values and personal choices of care.[33]

As laboratory science and the germ theory of disease took hold of the public imagination in the early 1900s—and mercury and bloodletting were on their way out—the public started to look toward regular doctors and surgeons with more respect. The American Medical Association took this opportunity to establish a Council on Medical Education in order to "upgrade medical education."[34] The council's goal was to close half the medical schools, thus halving the number of graduates and creating a more respected, higher-paid

---

31 "AMA History Timeline," American Medical Association, accessed May 6, 2015, www.ama-assn.org//ama/pub/about-ama/our-history/ama-history-timeline.page.

32 Harris L. Coulter, *Divided Legacy, Volume III: The Conflict Between Homeopathy and the American Medical Association* (Berkeley: North Atlantic Books, 1973).

33 Gerald E. Markowitz and David Karl Rosner, "Doctors in Crisis: A Study of the Use of Medical Education Reform to Establish Modern Professional Elitism in Medicine," *American Quarterly* 25, no. 1 (1973):83–107.

34 Dana Ullman, *The Homeopathic Revolution* (Berkeley: North Atlantic Books, 2007). The homeopaths at first supported this measure, because surveys in the American Medical Association's own journal (JAMA) showed that graduates of the conventional medical schools failed the national exams at nearly twice the rate as graduates of homeopathic colleges.

profession for physicians.[35] (Doctors, in those days, were often paid less than mechanics.[36])

It was a laudable goal, except that it still had a hint of hostility in it, as well as more than a whiff of elitism. AMA members had been complaining bitterly that their profession was overcrowded, and that they weren't getting enough respect, or enough money, because too many in their profession were of "coarse and common fiber."[37] The president of the AMA, in 1903, gave a speech that talked with disdain about night schools that allowed clerks, janitors, street-car conductors, and others employed during the day to earn a medical degree.[38]

"It is to be hoped that with higher standards universally applied, their number will soon be adequately reduced, and that only the fittest will survive," declared the editors of the *Journal of the American Medical Association*.[39] This sort of social Darwinism was typical of the era, and typical of the economic mind-set that says people perform better when they are forced to compete for limited resources.

In 1908, with funding from the Carnegie Foundation, the AMA's Council on Medical Education sent Abraham Flexner to do a survey of all US medical schools, and to provide a report on the quality of their teaching and other resources. (Two years earlier, the CME had already classified US medical schools into three groups: A = acceptable, B = doubtful, and C = unacceptable, and had shared this information with Flexner.[40]) When Flexner's report was published, it quickly became the basis of the AMA's campaign to standardize

35 Gerald E. Markowitz and David Karl Rosner, "Doctors in Crisis: A Study of the Use of Medical Education Reform to Establish Modern Professional Elitism in Medicine," *American Quarterly* 25, no. 1 (1973):83–107.
36 G. F. Shears, "Making a Choice," *Cosmopolitan*, April, 1903, 654.
37 Inez C. Philbrick, "Medical Colleges and Professional Standards," *JAMA* 36, no. 24 (1901).
38 "Medical Education," *Science* 17:763.
39 Andrew H. Beck, "Flexner Report and the Standardization of American Medical Education," *JAMA* 291, no. 17 (2004).
40 "AMA History Timeline," American Medical Association, accessed May 6, 2015, www.ama-assn.org//ama/pub/about-ama/our-history/ama-history-timeline.page.

medical education and close certain schools. Flexner recommended closing all of the nation's 151 medical schools, except for thirty-one that he had chosen.[41]

In 1912, a group of state licensing boards banded together and agreed to base their accreditation policies on standards determined by the AMA's council, and medical schools began rapidly closing down.[42] The next year, the AMA established a Propaganda Department whose task was to "gather and disseminate information concerning health fraud and quackery," and more schools were closed. By 1928, the Propaganda Department had been renamed the "Bureau of Investigation,"[43] a sharp signal to the remaining "nonregular" doctors that the AMA had clearly established itself— without ever having gotten permission from the government—as a national regulatory agency for the practice of medicine.

Several changes ensued, dramatically altering how medicine was defined and taught.

In 1900, the United States had a flourishing women's medical profession, with 7,000 female physicians (compared to 258 in England and 95 in France) who ran hospitals, taught in medical schools, and were deeply involved in important public health reforms.[44] After the AMA's council formed, six of the seven medical schools for women were shut down, resulting in a 33 percent reduction in female graduates.[45]

Fourteen medical schools for African-Americans had been established after slavery was abolished. Only seven remained, but on Flexner's recommendation, five of those were closed, leaving only

41 Barbara M. Barzansky and Norman Gevitz, *Beyond Flexner: Medical Education in the Twentieth Century* (Westport: Greenwood Press, 1992).

42 Gerald E. Markowitz and David Karl Rosner, "Doctors in Crisis: A Study of the Use of Medical Education Reform to Establish Modern Professional Elitism in Medicine," *American Quarterly* 25, no. 1 (1973) 83–107.

43 "AMA History Timeline," American Medical Association, accessed May 6, 2015, www.ama-assn.org//ama/pub/about-ama/our-history/ama-history-timeline.page.

44 Shari L. Barkin, et al., "Unintended Consequences of the Flexner Report: Women in Pediatrics" *Pediatrics* 126, no. 6 (2010):1055–57.

45 Paul Starr, *The Social Transformation of American Medicine* (New York: Basic, 1982), 124.

The Extinction of Medical Knowledge

Medical knowledge worldwide is at risk of extinction. As global companies disrupt ancient ecologies, and plant and animal species go extinct, so do the diverse languages, cultures, medical traditions, and pharmacological knowledge bases that coevolved with them. The loss of languages is profound, and escalating. UNESCO estimates that more than half of the world's 6,900 languages are in danger of extinction by the end of this century. Other researchers say that, on average, one language disappears every two weeks.[*,†,‡]

Historically, explorers, missionaries, and anthropologists documented native uses of herbs, but most of the texts they compiled lack the subtleties that someone actually wanting to use those herbs would need to know. It's not the list of plants that one needs, nor even the list of illnesses that each plant treats—it's the living, ongoing relationships between the practitioner, the herbs, the patient, and the landscape that form a whole system of indigenous health care.

Some traditional cultures harvest wild food and medicines the way they hunt animals: with caution not to change the conditions that the plants need in order to survive, nor to decimate the population by overharvesting. This kind of conscientiousness involves a deep relationship with the plants themselves, but also an understanding of the whole ecosystem and its natural changes over time.

When global economics comes into play, and entrepreneurs

---

[*] http://www.unesco.org/new/en/culture/themes/endangered-languages/. UNESCO also notes that 96 percent of the world's 6,000 languages are spoken by 4 percent of the world's population and 90 percent of the world's languages are not represented on the Internet.

[†] Thomas H. Maugh II, "Researchers Say a Language Disappears Every Two Weeks," *Los Angeles Times*, September 19, 2007.

[‡] Peter K. Austin and Julia Sallabank, Introduction to *Cambridge Handbook of Endangered Languages*, by Peter K. Austin and Julia Sallabank (Cambridge: Cambridge University Press, 2011).

seek to profit from the sale of herbs that they themselves don't depend on for health, they often overlook the question of long-term local sustainability. For example, someone looking to make a quick buck may have little understanding of the history and needs of a stand of trees that have provided medicinal bark for a small group of villagers for thousands of years.

In 2010, the *Times of India* reported that 93 percent of the nearly 400 wild herbs used in Ayurvedic medicine are endangered because of habitat loss and overharvesting. The herb companies are just the tip of the iceberg, however. Cultivation of monocultures like corn, soybeans, cotton, coffee, and sugarcane, and factors such as deforestation and climate change, all put pressures on the complex web of relationships needed to sustain the wild pharmacy that used to cover every part of the globe.

Medical diversity suffers in other ways as Western science takes over the global imagination, and East, West, North, and South all start to move toward a monolithic view. Over a period of several years in the late 1950s, a small committee of scientists in the People's Republic of China condensed 3,000 years of diverse family and local traditions of herbal medicine and acupuncture into a small set of textbooks leaning heavily on Western scientific terminology (which then became the foundation of acupuncture education worldwide) and dared to call this new condensed version of medicine "Traditional Chinese Medicine." [*,†]

---

[*] Certain niches of medical diversity survive, often due to circumstances as random as those that preserve niches of biodiversity. The unique forms of acupuncture practiced in Japan were nearly outlawed after World War II, until someone pointed out that acupuncture was, essentially, a form of welfare for the visually impaired. Acupuncture is traditionally a profession for the blind in Japan, and if acupuncture were outlawed, they would be dependent on their families or the state for income. So the new law was changed: and for a time, only blind people were allowed to practice acupuncture in Japan. This preserved a unique style of acupuncture during a time of rapid modernization.

[†] Kim Taylor, *Chinese Medicine in Early Communist China, 1945–63: A Medicine of Revolution* (London: Psychology Press, 2005).

two.[46] Flexner's report had also suggested a limited role for African-American physicians, portraying them as useful only "to treat their own race." (Echoes of that thinking persist today, though in subtler language.) His view of their role was not primarily as physicians but as teachers of hygiene and sanitation to prevent African-American diseases from spreading to white populations, as he portrayed African-Americans as a source of "infection and contagion."[47]

Most of the Southern and Midwestern rural medical schools that were not connected to universities with large endowments were also closed, as were the affordable night schools that were open to poor and working-class medical students.[48,49] Holistic and preventive forms of medicine were no longer taught in medical schools, and states began passing laws that prevented naturopathic and other "nonregular" physicians from practicing medicine. The mechanistic, rather than the ecological, view of the body, and reductionist laboratory science, became the required basis of medical school curriculum and medical licensing exams.[50]

Under intense pressure from the new "medical profession," state after state passed laws outlawing midwifery and restricting the practice of obstetrics to doctors, even though studies were showing that doctors had far less understanding of the birth process than traditional midwives. This made obstetric and gynecological care too expensive for most poor and working-class women.[51]

Finally, the Rockefeller Institute created a system by which

---

46 Earl H. Harley, "The Forgotten History of Defunct Black Medical Schools in the 19th and 20th Centuries and the Impact of the Flexner Report," *Journal of the National Medical Association*, 98, no. 9 (2006):1425–29.

47 Louis W Sullivan, MD, and Ilana Suez Mittman, PhD, "The State of Diversity in the Health Professions a Century After Flexner," *Academic Medicine* 85, no. 2 (2010):246–53.

48 Andrew H. Beck, "Flexner Report and the Standardization of American Medical Education," *JAMA* 291, no. 17 (2004).

49 Gerald E. Markowitz and David Karl Rosner, "Doctors in Crisis: A Study of the Use of Medical Education Reform to Establish Modern Professional Elitism in Medicine," *American Quarterly* 25, no. 1 (1973):83–107.

50 Ibid.

51 Barbara Ehrenreich, *Witches, Midwives, and Nurses: A History of Women Healers* (New York: The Feminist Press at CUNY, 1973).

medical research grants had to be vetted by a board of experts, primarily from the elite East Coast medical schools. (The first president of the institute was Flexner himself.) This led to more narrowing of the focus of medicine, and to further closings, isolation, and impoverishment of Southern and Western medical institutions that depended on state funding rather than on wealthy benefactors.[52]

The combined result of all these changes made the next wave of doctors—who went on to become the next wave of medical school professors—primarily white, wealthy, competitive men who excelled at linear thinking. Our current system, with all its marvelous progress and its quirky flaws, was designed, taught, and developed by them.

So what went missing? What would our medical system look like if it had not been streamlined in the quest for higher profits? What would it look like if it had also been designed, taught, and developed by women, by people of color, by people interested in a variety of holistic systems-based approaches, and by people who had grown up in poor and working-class households?

We only know one part of the answer: "*Not like this.*"

Parallels between Industrial Agriculture and Industrial Medicine

As I have sought to understand the issues of our current health-care system, I have noticed parallels between agriculture and medicine, particularly in the ways they have adapted to the larger markets of the modern-day growth economy.

In both realms, we have shifted away from what I've been calling

52 Gerald E. Markowitz and David Karl Rosner, "Doctors in Crisis: A Study of the Use of Medical Education Reform to Establish Modern Professional Elitism in Medicine," *American Quarterly* 25, no. 1 (1973):83–107.

a "fertile" model, and toward a more "sterile" one that competes with—or kills off—whatever is not wanted. We turned away from stewardship, collaboration, and cooperatives, and toward competition, profits, and patenting. We chose pesticides and herbicides, rubber gloves and antibiotics, and turned away from compost and manure, human touch and probiotics. Both agriculture and medicine shifted from seeing things in the context of whole integrated systems, focusing instead on individual parts. We moved away from diversity and overlapping functions, and focused instead on specialization, standardization, and monocropping. We abandoned small-scale localized infrastructure and invested in large-scale corporations. In the process, we lost touch with traditional knowledge that works with natural patterns and cycles, and rushed instead into chemical and high-tech manipulation of nature. This has left us with a planet swimming in industrial waste and struggling to adapt to a changing climate—all under the guise of feeding ourselves and keeping ourselves healthy.

Biomechanistic Puzzles

The industrial farming model—in which we put an animal in a box, away from its natural environment, give it antibiotics and hormones, and then try to determine what nutrients it needs to be maximally productive; or put a seed into "sterilized" dirt, kill off all the weeds and bugs with chemicals, then try to figure out what artificial fertilizer the seed needs to be maximally productive—is strangely similar to the industrial medical model. We tend to look at a patient, like we look at the cow or the grain, as if he were a biomechanistic puzzle. We put him in a private room, away from natural influences, and give him industrially manufactured food and medicine with the goal of keeping him alive and functional for as long as possible.

It's not a bad goal, just an odd way of getting there, as the industrial approach doesn't take into account its effect on everything outside of the hospital. Nor does it take into account the effect on the psyches of the people who work there. Almost 50 percent of doctors report symptoms of burnout.[53,54]

Industrial models of agriculture and medicine are characterized by:

- Human manipulation of nature
- Machines, speed, and technology
- Isolating parts to understand the whole
- Killing off "bugs" with pesticides or antibiotics
- Laboratory knowledge
- Monocropping and specialization
- Privacy
- Experts doling out information to those who can pay
- Simple chemical fertilizers and synthetic vitamins
- "Sterility" and separation from the natural environment
- Large, centralized farms and hospitals
- Economic growth and profits as the primary definition of success
- Extraction of resources
- Focusing on problems in order to sell solutions
- Global production of supplies

The Loss of Resiliency

As more and more technology is available to separate us from anything that is uncomfortable, unwanted, inconvenient, or that we simply don't know how to deal with, we become less and less resilient.

Resiliency is the ability to rebound after challenges and to respond and adapt to changing circumstances. It is the hallmark of

53 Tait D. Shanafelt, et al., "Burnout and Satisfaction with Work-Life Balance Among US Physicians Relative to the General US Population," *Archives of Internal Medicine* 172, no. 18 (October 8, 2012):1377–85.
54 David Bornstein, "Medicine's Search for Meaning," *New York Times*, September 18, 2013.

all species that share the resources of the Earth. None of us would be here if we weren't resilient. Diversity and complexity help to make systems resilient, flexible, and adaptable, yet those are precisely the qualities that our modern systems of medicine and agriculture have left behind.

Our over-reliance on technology to control the complexity around us teaches us just the opposite: that we don't have to shift or adapt or compromise. Instead we can take a drug, change a genetic code, or "surgically remove" whatever is in our way—whether it is a lump of fat tissue on our belly, an insect eating our corn, or a group of people who live on land we want for mining purposes.

The idea of isolating parts, which has guided most scientific pursuits, has also allowed us to imagine that we can isolate our own health from the health of our environment.

One could forget, in a twenty-minute consult with a patient, while sitting indoors, that health is much larger than the body. One could forget, while talking to a cancer patient, that the incinerators of medical waste have until recently been one of the major causes of cancer-causing dioxins in the environment.[55] One could forget, when writing a prescription for a middle-age man for a cholesterol-lowering drug, that the pharmaceuticals you prescribe are peed out and persist in the water table, where they act as reproductive inhibitors for the swans and loons, porcupines and otters that all live near waterways.[56]

One could forget that the antipsychotic you prescribe for one patient persists in the "purified" drinking water of the next patient— creating interesting side effects for those drinking from a city water system.[57] One could forget that if Inuit mothers living far from any

55 Joe Thornton, et al. "Hospitals and Plastics. Dioxin Prevention and Medical Waste Incinerators," *Public Health Reports* 111, no. 4 (July–August 1996):298–313.
56 C. G. Daughton, "The Environmental Life Cycle of Pharmaceuticals," illustration, US EPA, NRL (Las Vegas, NV: December 2006), www.epa.gov/esd/bios/daughton/drug-lifecycle.pdf.
57 Ibid.

factories have high levels of pollutants in their breast milk,[58] then the pregnant mother in front of you can't protect her health just by getting enough sleep, eating well, and exercising—she is part of an unhealthy system.

When we change the biology around us, the chemistry around us, the genetics around us, and even the physics around us, we change the natural systems we rely on for health and survival. As we begin to fathom the interconnectedness of life, the doctor's mandate "first, do no harm" becomes a much more complex task.

How do we adapt our forms of caring for one another to take all these aspects into account?

The Fertile Model of Care

"In nature there is no 'above' and 'below,' and there are no hierarchies. There are only networks nesting within other networks."
—Fritjof Capra[59]

We stand at a crossroads, a unique point in time when we have:

- Huge technological knowledge that is still unfolding
- Vast traditional knowledge that is quickly disappearing
- Still relatively plentiful (though shrinking) resources

We are perhaps the only generation that has access to so many options. As we move forward, what kinds of solutions do we choose? Do we throw out everything we have learned and go back to the past? Do we grasp for yet another quick technological fix? Where should we look as we try to create the conditions for a healthy, resilient future?

---

58 Marla Cone, *Silent Snow: The Slow Poisoning of the Arctic* (New York: Grove Press, 2005).

59 Fritjof Capra, *The Web of Life* (New York: Anchor, 1977), 35.

Ecology has long known that the most fertile, vibrant place is at the "edge." The spaces where woods meet fields, and where rivers meet meadows, find themselves leaping with life. We are in one of those spaces now in the "ecology" of our understanding.

The Beauty of the Edge

Farmers and scientists working within the organic, permaculture, and regenerative agriculture movements have already questioned the long-term workability of large-scale industrialized agriculture. Out of these concerns have arisen many new integrated models that work with natural patterns and flows and revive traditional wisdom without necessarily abandoning technology altogether. These methods produce healthier, more resilient crops and animals that actually enrich the landscape—bringing water, lush plants, and biodiversity back to depleted land and brittle deserts. I think medicine is ready to do the same with our inner landscapes.

To do so means that we must acknowledge our place as one of many species living within—and dependent upon—a healthy functioning whole. We evolved out of the same natural cycles, patterns, and events as the other species around us, and we struggle with many of the same challenges. Plants and animals deal with bacterial, viral, fungal, and genetic illnesses just as we do. They need nutrients and clean water, and they rely on a wide variety of beneficial microorganisms for survival, just as we do. When they are resilient, they adapt and change and evolve, just as we do.

Given these parallels, we can adopt strategies for taking care of our inner landscapes and growing healthy people by observing the ways that sustainable agriculture, permaculture, and holistic land management take care of the outer landscape to grow healthy plants and animals.

Parallels between Regenerative Agriculture and Ecological Medicine

Ecological models of health care and agriculture are characterized by:

- Complexity and diversity
- Working with natural patterns and cycles
- Contextual understandings
- Complex nutrients from natural sources
- Creating conditions for self-organizing systems
- Boosting natural immunity and resiliency
- Using natural predators and microorganisms to balance ecosystems inside and outside the body
- Collaboration and cooperatives
- Networks of shared information and support
- Multipurposed stacking of functions
- Small, localized, easily accessible producers and providers integrated into the community and landscape
- Participation in regenerative systems, "cradle to cradle"
- Stewardship, rather than ownership
- Alliances between species and participation in the ecosystem
- Use of the Precautionary Principle before accepting new technologies[60]
- Integration of traditional knowledge and indigenous ways of knowing along with creative use of technology
- A slow and steady pace, and long-term connections

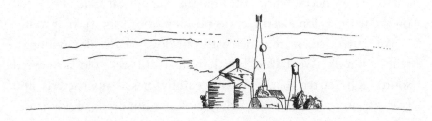

60 See the section on wild law in chapter 10 for more on the precautionary principle.

CHAPTER TWO

Ancient Relationships: Beyond the Germ Theory of Disease

"Bacteria are not germs, but the germinators—and fabric—of all life on Earth. In declaring war on them we declared war on the underlying living structure of the planet—on all life-forms we can see—on ourselves."

—Stephen Harrod Buhner[1]

"Just how dirty is Hygeia?"

—James Hillman[2]

When my children were young, our chickens walked in and out of the house; I wiped up accidents if they occurred, but I didn't scrub with Lysol. The boys played outside in the dirt and mud in the summer and swam in the river every day instead of taking showers. In winter, they bathed once or twice a week, whether they needed it or not. I taught them to eat food after it fell on the floor, as long as there was nothing obviously sticking to it.

We shared ice cream cones with our dog. We drank raw unpasteurized milk. We baked bread from a 200-year-old fermented sourdough starter that had purposefully picked up bacteria and yeasts from the unwashed kitchen tables of hundreds of women in

---

1   Stephen Harrod Buhner, *The Lost Language of Plants: The Ecological Importance of Plant Medicines for Life on Earth* (White River Junction, VT: Chelsea Green, 2002).
2   Quoted by Jeannine Parvati in *Hygieia: A Woman's Herbal* (Freestone Collective, 1978).

log cabins across the American prairies and huts across the steppes of Russia.

Was this living dangerously? I don't think so.

Our Microscopic Allies

"The pathogen is nothing, the terrain is everything."
—Claude Bernard

"Bernard was right, the terrain is everything."
—Louis Pasteur's dying words

The most basic allies that we have overlooked in the era of industrial medicine are so close to us we can't even see them. Our focus on sterility has made us blind. Modern medicine is just beginning to rediscover and celebrate the secret of life, something that regenerative agriculture has already embraced: a thriving microbial ecosystem.

Each one of us harbors an ecosystem that includes at least 1,000 trillion bacteria and other microorganisms. Ninety percent of the cells in our bodies are not our own. Yet for years and years we have associated "germs" with illness, and have done everything we could to get rid of our germs: scrubbing furiously at our bodies, inside and out, with antiseptic wipes and antibiotic regimens, and purifying our food chain so that no one else's germs can enter us. And it's true: when someone's immune system is compromised—because of a virus, because of a cut in the skin or membranes, or because of stress or malnutrition—there are a few strains of bacteria (fewer than 200) that will opportunistically come in and create an infection; sometimes a horrendous infection. But most of the time, *most* bacteria create health—lush, complicated, life-giving, fertile health—in our bodies, in the soil, in the ocean, and everywhere around us. That's because bacteria and other microorganisms help things grow and thrive, including us.

Building Healthy Inner Landscapes

It was once believed that babies were sterile at birth, but it turns out that even in the protected space of the uterus, fetuses start to develop a microbiome: an ecological community of microorganisms that literally share a person's body space.[3]

As soon as infants are out in the world, they need many more beneficial bacteria in order to survive. They pick up some of those healthy bacteria (such as *Bifidobacteria* and *Lactobacillus*) from the birth canal, which colonize their digestive tracts and allow them to easily digest breast milk. These lay the groundwork for other helpful gut bacteria to be welcomed in through breastfeeding (breast milk has more than 600 species of bacteria[4,5]) and casual contact, such as sucking on fingers, toys, and everything around them. The skin of babies is colonized with bacteria via similar routes: first the birth canal, and then by contact with the skin of people who care for them—all teeming with microorganisms.

Traditionally, after weaning, children and adults constantly replenished their intestines with beneficial microorganisms by eating raw fruits and vegetables with minuscule bits of soil still clinging to them, raw milk products (from healthy, grass-fed cows), raw or rare fish and meats, and a wide array of lacto-fermented foods full of beneficial bacteria and yeasts.[6] Once mobile, we travel in a personal cloud of microorganisms, extending out from our bodies into the air around us, that announces our arrival wherever we go, leaves traces of our travels on surfaces around us, and mingles momentarily with other people's clouds as we wait in line for school lunches.

3   Ylva Kai-Larsen, et al., "A Review of the Innate Immune Defense of the Human Foetus and Newborn, with the Emphasis on Antimicrobial Peptides," *Acta Paediatrica* 103, no. 10 (2014):1000–08.
4   Katherine M Hunt, et al., "Characterization of the Diversity and Temporal Stability of Bacterial Communities in Human Milk," *PLOS One* 6, no. 10 (2011).
5   E. A. Quinn, "Human Milk Has a Microbiome—And the Bacteria Are Protecting Mothers and Infants!" *Biomarkers & Milk*, December 14, 2014.
6   Sandor Ellix Katz, *Wild Fermentation: The Flavor, Nutrition, and Craft of Live-Culture Foods* (White River Junction, VT: Chelsea Green, 2003).

The landscape of microorganisms in our guts, mouths, noses, eyes, ears, genitalia, skin, and personal space is built up gradually, and then replenished throughout life from the microbiomes of people and animals we touch and kiss, foods we eat, and the world around us.

By adulthood, each of us has a uniquely personal microbiome reflecting not just our mother's microbiota, but also the personal history of each of the people who have held us and cared for us; the dogs, cats, and cows who have licked us; the friends we have wrestled with; the foods we have eaten; the cities we have lived in and traveled to; the people with whom we have shared intimate moments or passed on a crowded street; the money and objects we have touched; and the places where we dug in the dirt, swam in the river, chewed on the grass, or ate wild strawberries.

Life, when lived as it is meant to be lived, is a deeply communal activity. It's a sensual dance of species through spaces, the seen and unseen, a continual weaving together of our interior and exterior worlds.

Lacto-Fermented Foods

Long before the Industrial Revolution, before anyone tried feeding whiskey swill to cows, people understood how to partner with microorganisms to do work. In particular, they knew how to preserve foods, extract nutrients, change flavors, and prevent illnesses with special help from a family of bacteria called *Lactobacilli*, along with yeasts and other tiny allies.

Traditionally cured lacto-fermented meats, such as salami, can hang from the rafters for months without going bad, with no need for the addition of nitrates or nitrites (which have been linked to a variety of cancers). Scurvy on long voyages was conquered by Captain James Cook, who stocked his ships with barrels of live, bubbling sauerkraut, and Polynesian seafarers sustained themselves on long voyages with fermented taro root, called Poi. Korean families buried cabbages and turnips—flavored with garlic, ginger, shrimp, and hot peppers—in containers underground in order to be able to have enzyme-rich vegetables in the form of kimchi all winter. The Swiss made cheese out of bacterially rich unpasteurized milk and cream during the spring and summer months (when the cows were grazing on fast-growing pastures) and ate it all winter to replenish themselves with nutrients.[7]

Traditional methods of pickling vegetables and curing meats all depend on bacteria, as does the production of traditional beer, mead, wine, root beer, and ginger ale. (In fact, these are the food production processes that Louis Pasteur was studying in order to understand how bacteria work, before he invented new methods of preservation that involved killing off pathogenic bacteria rather than working with natural food-preserving qualities of beneficial bacteria.) Ketchup, chutney, sauerkraut, relish, salsa, and most of the steak sauces we enjoy were originally made with the help of beneficial bacteria, as well. We still crave these flavors, but today's versions no longer carry any of the original health-giving benefits.

In our modern diets, we pasteurize our pickles and sauerkraut, preserve our pepperoni with nitrites and nitrates, irradiate our meat and many vegetables, and overcook many of the other fresh foods that we traditionally would rely on for beneficial bacteria.

Until recently, yogurt was one of the only lacto-fermented foods that managed to survive the industrialization of our food system. But even yogurt, when produced in industrial facilities, has only a fraction of the types of beneficial bacteria it would have if it were made in people's homes from raw milk.

---

7   Ron Schmidt, *The Untold Story of Milk: Green Pastures, Contented Cows, and Raw Dairy Foods* (Washington, DC: New Trends Publishing, 2003).

Health Benefits of Fermented Foods

Fermentation guru Sandor Ellix Katz writes about some of the research on health aspects of fermented foods in his book *Wild Fermentation*:[8,9]

- Eating live fermented foods directly supplies your digestive tract with living cultures essential to breaking down food and assimilating nutrients, preventing diarrhea and dysentery, and improving infant survival rates.[10]
- Ferments can inhibit growth of pathogenic bacteria, such as *E.coli, Salmonella, Staphylococcus aureus,* and *Shigella*.[11]
- A study in the journal *Nutrition* concluded that *Lactobacilli* compete with potential pathogens for receptor sites at the mucosal cell surfaces of the intestines, providing a sort of "ecoimmunonutrition."[12]
- Fermentation creates new nutrients. As they go through their life cycles, microbial cultures create B vitamins, including folic acid, riboflavin, niacin, thiamin, and biotin.
- Once they are residing in the large intestine, these bacteria also produce essential vitamins—K, B_{12}, thiamine, and riboflavin—that human bodies cannot produce by themselves.

8   Sandor Ellix Katz, *Wild Fermentation: The Flavor, Nutrition, and Craft of Live-Culture Foods* (White River Junction, VT: Chelsea Green, 2003).
9   Hundreds more research studies can be found in the book *The Life Bridge: The Way to Longevity with Probiotic Nutrients* (New Chapter, 2002).
10 Wilbald Lorri and Ulf Svanberg, "Lower Prevalence of Diarrhoea in Young Children Fed Lactic Acid-Fermented Cereal Gruels," *Food and Nutrition Bulletin* 15, no. 1 (1994):57–63.
11 S. K. Mbuguaa and J. Njenga, "The Antimicrobial Activity of Fermented Uji," *Ecology of Food and Nutrition* 15, no. 3 (1992):191–98.
12 S. Bengmark, "Immunonutrition: Role of Biosurfactants, Fiber, and Probiotic Bacteria," Nutrition 14, nos. 7–8 (1998):585–94.

- *Lactobacilli* create omega-3 fatty acids, essential for cell membrane and immune function.
- Fermentation removes toxins, such as cyanide, from otherwise-inedible foods like certain varieties of cassava. It also removes lesser toxins like phytic acid from grains, which would otherwise interfere with absorption of minerals.
- Fermentation breaks down nutrients into more easily digestible forms. Tempeh and miso are more digestible than soybeans, and yogurt and cheese are often more digestible than milk. Sourdough breads are more digestible than breads made with baker's yeast.
- The UN Food and Agriculture Organization actively promotes fermentation as a critical source of nutrients worldwide because it improves the bioavailability of minerals present in food.

If lacto-fermented foods are so good for us, why aren't they widely available in supermarkets? It has to do with profits. Lacto-fermented foods are alive and often literally bursting with enzymatic energy. Jars can break or overflow because of the fizzy aliveness of ferments. Like wine, batches of lacto-fermented foods also vary in flavor depending on which yeasts and bacteria are floating around in the air on a certain day, and depending on the temperature, season, and region they are made in. A live pickle (made by putting a cucumber in brine and letting it create its own vinegar, not by sticking a cucumber in vinegar) will taste very different if you eat it on day 6 versus day 20 or day 40.

None of these are benefits if you are trying to create a brand-name product that always tastes the same and can be shipped all over the country and stored for months, or even years, on shelves without refrigeration. To sell things on a large scale means they must be easy to transport, have a long shelf life, and be predictable in flavor so that you can create a brand name that people "trust."

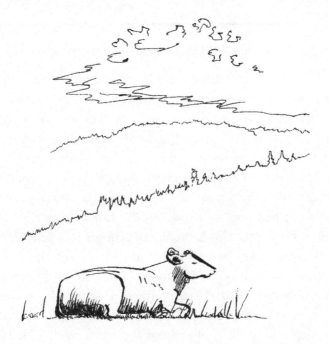

Dirty Rats, Vaginal Births, "Old Friends," and the Hygiene Hypothesis

In 1989, scientists proposed that the rate of chronic illness—in particular, allergic and autoimmune disorders—was rising in wealthier developed nations because of a lack of exposure to dirt and bacteria, specifically in the early years when the immune system is developing. This theory was nicknamed the "hygiene hypothesis." It started with one famous study, published in the *Lancet*, which showed that babies growing up on farms who were exposed to stables and to raw milk had a lower incidence of asthma and allergies,[13] and another study that showed that children who had taken antibiotics in infancy were more likely to develop asthma.[14]

---

13 J. Riedler, et al., "Exposure to Farming in Early Life and Development of Asthma and Allergy: A Cross-Sectional Survey," *Lancet* 358, no. 9288 (2001):1129–33.

14 Fawziah Marra, et al., "Does Antibiotic Exposure During Infancy Lead to Development of Asthma?: A Systematic Review and Metaanalysis," National Center for Biotechnology Information," *Chest* 129, no. 3 (2006):610–18.

Traditional Wisdom about the Microbiome

For 2,500 years, Chinese medicine has taught that three of the body's seemingly disparate areas—the respiratory system, the large intestines, and the skin—are all part of one system, the *wei qi* or "protective function," that regulates grief and depression and modulates immunity.

Traditional Chinese dietary therapy also taught that people with weakness of this protective function could be nourished best by eating foods with a "rotten" flavor. We puzzled over this language in acupuncture school, but it became clear once I understood the health benefits of lacto-fermented foods. The more I learn about the interaction between "rotten" lacto-fermented foods, the microbiome, mood regulation, and immunity, the more I appreciate the depth of traditional wisdom and "kitchen medicine."

The Chinese theory is absolutely correct:

- The skin (including orifices), the mucosal membranes of the respiratory system, and the large intestine are precisely the areas of the body where the microbiome is most active.
- The microbiome can be nourished with "rotten" lacto-fermented foods.
- Both mood and immunity, if not properly regulated by a well-nourished microbiome, can easily go awry.

Wild rats, whether living in the countryside or in city sewers, were also found to have healthier immune systems than laboratory rats raised without exposure to germs and dirt.[15] The explanation

15 Ashley M Trama, et al., "Lymphocyte Phenotypes in Wild-Caught Rats Suggest Potential Mechanisms Underlying Increased Immune Sensitivity in Post-Industrial Environments," *Cellular & Molecular Immunology* 9, no. 2 (2012):163–74.

given was that the dirty rats' rough and rugged immune systems were better poised to fight actual pathogens, rather than reacting over mild irritants the way sheltered immune systems do when they have no actual work to do.

In our highly sterilized world, autoimmune and allergic disorders are on the rise. One in every 12 people in the US now has asthma (and 1 in 6 African-American children).[16] The National Institutes of Health says the prevalence of autoimmune diseases, such as multiple sclerosis, type 1 diabetes, and inflammatory bowel disorders, is rising dramatically, as well. It now appears that the *lack* of certain gut bacteria (as well as lack of other gut inhabitants, like worms[17]) is implicated.

Babies born by cesarean section miss out on the initial colonizing bacteria from the mother's birth canal and perineum—and have 20 percent higher incidence of childhood asthma and a decrease in overall immunity.[18,19] This puts a sting in the fact that the current rate of C-sections in the US is climbing fast—about one-third of all births in the US are now C-sections (and half of all births in China). The World Health Organization estimates that only about 15 percent of these C-sections are necessary.[20]

One-quarter of babies born in the United States are never breastfed, and half are breastfed for less than six months,[21] which represents a gigantic blow to a baby's immune system at birth.

---

16 "Asthma in the US," Centers for Disease Control and Prevention, accessed May 27, 2015, http://www.cdc.gov/VitalSigns/asthma/.

17 Y. Osada and T. Kanazawa, "Parasitic Helminths: New Weapons Against Immunological Disorders," *J Biomed Biotechnol* (2010):743–58.

18 S. Thavagnanam, et al., "A Meta-analysis of the Association Between Caesarean Section and Childhood Asthma," *Clinical & Experimental Allergy* 38, no. 4 (2007):629–33.

19 Anu Huurre, et al., "Mode of Delivery: Effects on Gut Microbiota and Humoral Immunity," *Neonatology* 93, no. 4 (2008):236–40.

20 Denise Grady, "Caesarean Births Are at a High in US," *New York Times*, March 23, 2010.

21 "Breastfeeding Report Card," Centers for Disease Control and Prevention, accessed May 13, 2015, http://www.cdc.gov/breastfeeding/data/reportcard.htm.

There is no passive immunity from the mother without breast milk and the hundreds of varieties of good bacteria it provides.[22]

Graham Rook, a professor at the Centre for Infectious Diseases and International Health in London, renamed the hygiene hypothesis the "Old Friends Hypothesis." The problem, according to Rook, is not so much about being too clean; it's that in our newly sterilized lives we are missing out on many important members of our inner ecosystem, with which we coevolved, and that we actually rely on to *teach* our system how to respond without overreacting—to the environment, to food, to events, and to its own tissues.[23,24]

Mood-Altering Bugs

Gut bacteria influence our behavior and thinking, our movements and moods. Using gene signaling, Swedish scientists were able to show that the brain chemicals serotonin and dopamine—as well as synapse function in general—all appear to be regulated by colonizing bacteria, and that learning, memory, and motor control were all affected by the absence of gut bacteria.

Mice raised in germ-free environments exhibit different behaviors than those raised with normal microorganisms. When microorganisms were reintroduced to the germ-free mice early in life they would exhibit "normal" behavior, but not if the microorganisms were introduced later.[25,26] Other studies showed that by transplanting gut bacteria from a group of mice known to be more passive to another, more active group, they were able to predictably

22 Lars A. Hanson, "Breastfeeding Provides Passive and Likely Long-Lasting Active Immunity," *Annals of Allergy, Asthma & Immunology* 81, no. 6 (1998):523–33, 537.
23 Graham A. W. Rook, "Review Series on Helminths, Immune Modulation and the Hygiene Hypothesis: The Broader Implications of the Hygiene Hypothesis," *Immunology* 126 (2009):3–11.
24 Graham A. W. Rook, et al., "Microbial 'Old Friends,' Immunoregulation and Stress Resilience," *Evolution, Medicine, and Public Health*, no. 1 (2013):46–64.
25 McMaster University, "Gut Bacteria Linked to Behavior: That Anxiety May Be in Your Gut, Not in Your Head," *Science Daily*, May 17, 2011.
26 Emmanuel Denou, et al., "The Intestinal Microbiota Determines Mouse Behavior and Brain BDNF Levels." *Gastroenterology* 141, no. 2 (2011):599–609.

change the mice's behavior, and vice versa.[27] Our little friends in our bellies apparently have a lot of opinions.

So what else are we missing when we have cesareans, bottle-feed our babies, bathe them every day, feed them baby foods out of a jar, and give them antibiotics "just in case"? Studies have linked deficiencies and imbalances of gut bacteria (particularly in the first few months of life) to depression, anxiety, autism, and other brain disorders, as well as to allergic and autoimmune disorders, and disturbances in gastrointestinal, metabolic, neuroendocrine, circulatory, and immune functions. The gut microbiota also influence drug metabolism and toxicity, dietary calorific bioavailability, immune system conditioning and response, and postsurgical recovery.[28,29,30,31]

The most striking part of this is that our human DNA is actually incomplete without the proper bacterial companions. Our DNA leaves the responsibility for some developmental jobs to the DNA of the bacteria it assumes will take up residency soon after birth. And not just minor jobs. Over the course of evolution, the colonization of the gut by microorganisms in early infancy appears to have become *part of the process of brain development*, which changes behavior and brain functioning later in life.[32,33] Likewise, our

27 Ibid.
28 James M. Kinross, Ara W. Darzi, & Jeremy K. Nicholson, "Gut Microbiome-Host Interactions in Health and Disease," *Genome Medicine* 3, no. 3 (2011).
29 Timothy G. Dinan, et al., "Collective Unconscious: How Gut Microbes Shape Human Behavior," *Journal of Psychiatric Research* 63 (2015):1–9.
30 Moises Velasquez-Manoff, "An Immune Disorder at the Root of Autism," *New York Times*, August 26, 2012.
31 Charles L. Raison, et al., "Inflammation, Sanitation, and Consternation: Loss of Contact with Coevolved, Tolerogenic Microorganisms and the Pathophysiology and Treatment of Major Depression," *Archives of General Psychiatry* 67, no. 12 (2010):1211–24.
32 Rochellys Diaz Heijtz, et al., "Normal Gut Microbiota Modulates Brain Development and Behavior," *PNAS* (2011):3047–52.
33 Tolerance is one of three ways we learn to deal with potential pathogens. The first is avoidance (like seeing someone with a snotty nose and deciding not to kiss them). The second is by attacking a pathogen (which is what our immune system does as it creates most of the symptoms we think of as colds, flus, allergies, infections; coughing, fevers, runny noses, swelling, etc.). The third is to develop a tolerance to the pathogen: to learn to live with it or let it pass through us without being harmed by it.

My Mother Doesn't Want to Eat Worms

My mother doesn't want to eat worms.

I explain to her that although they are alive, these particular worms I am recommending won't reproduce inside of her, and that if she needed to, she could kill them off with a single dose of worming medicine. In the meantime, she could stop her autoimmune disorder in its tracks. Autoimmune disorders, such as asthma, multiple sclerosis, ulcerative colitis, and Crohn's disease, are all significantly lessened by the presence of parasitic worms in the intestines—to the extent that some doctors are actually repopulating patients with worms in order to improve symptoms.[*,†,‡]

She's not convinced. She shudders. But she is also desperate for a solution. Her own immune system is attacking her mucus membranes—giving her dry eyes and a dry mouth that keep her awake at night, and weight loss of five pounds a month. She is down to 110 pounds.

"How does it work again?" she asks.

"People and other animals evolved to have a few worms in them, just like the soil has worms. It's part of our inner ecosystem. The immune system expects them to be there, is ready for them, and is designed to keep them from getting out of hand. If you get dewormed as a child, the part of your immune system that is supposed to keep your gut's worm population at a healthy level has nothing to do, and no one to keep in check. So it starts attacking whatever other fleshy structures it can find: your own body's tissues. When you repopulate your intestines with just a few worms, your autoimmune system stops attacking your body and turns its attention back to the worms."

"It makes sense," she says. "But I'm just not there yet."

[*]   Y. Osada and T. Kanazawa, "Parasitic Helminths: New Weapons Against Immunological Disorders," *Journal of Biomedicine and Biotechnology*, 2010:743–58.

[†]   Mathilde Versini, et al., "Unraveling the Hygiene Hypothesis of Helminthes and Autoimmunity: Origins, Pathophysiology, and Clinical Applications," *BMC Medicine* 2015, 13:81.

[‡]   C. M. Finlay, et al. "Induction of Regulatory Cells by Helminth Parasites: Exploitation for the Treatment of Inflammatory Diseases," *Immunological Reviews*, No. 259 (2014):206–30.

DNA leaves some of the development of our immune system up to interactions with the collective genome of the microorganisms that, until recently, all humans hosted: our microbiome.[34] In other words? We wouldn't be humans without our worms and germs. Our DNA itself entrusts much of our survival to our willingness to host these tiny companions.

Dirty Little Secrets?

Canning factories aren't the only thing that has kept us at a distance from our bacterial allies. The soil that commercial vegetables are grown in also has lost many of its beneficial bacteria because of the use of tillage, long periods without plant cover, chemical fertilizers, herbicides, fungicides, and pesticides, all of which tend to interfere with soil microorganisms.

Just as beneficial bacteria help to make nutrients available to us in our digestive tracts, soil organisms are responsible for making minerals biologically available to plants.[35,36] Although various arguments circle around about the exact reasons why, researchers agree that average nutrient contents (including protein, calcium, phosphorus, iron, riboflavin, and vitamin C) of most vegetables and fruits have declined dramatically in the past fifty to seventy years.[37] Loss of soil microorganisms and their capacity to make nutrients available to plants may well be part of the issue. But it is more complicated than that.

34 S. K. Mazmanian, et al., "A Microbial Symbiosis Factor Prevents Intestinal Inflammatory Disease," *Nature* 453 (2008):620–25.

35 Elaine Ingham, Soil Carbon Workshops and Keynote Lecture at the Northeast Organic Farming Association Summer Conference, Amherst, Massachusetts, August 8–10, 2014.

36 "Dirt Poor: Have Fruits and Vegetables Become Less Nutritious?" http://www. scientificamerican.com/article/soil-depletion-and-nutrition-loss/.

37 Donald R. Davis, "Declining Fruit and Vegetable Nutrient Composition: What Is the Evidence?" *Horticultural Science* 44, no. 1 (February 2009):15–19.

Glyphosate, or Roundup®, is used as an herbicide on most GMO crops and as a drying agent on many others, but it was originally patented as a descalant to clean out mineral residues in industrial pipes and boilers—it does this by binding to minerals. This same chelating effect binds minerals in the soil when glyphosate is applied to crops. Monsanto patented it as an herbicide, then patented it again as a broad-spectrum antibacterial, in hopes of having it approved for medical use. It appears that it may be having an effect on our gut bacteria, as well.

Glyphosate's antibacterial properties take effect by creating mutations in the bacteria, not by killing them off directly. Glyphosate does this by inhibiting the "shikimate" pathway—an ancient metabolic pathway found in bacteria, algae, fungi, and plants (unless they have been genetically modified to be resistant to glyphosate's effects), but not in animals. By inhibiting this pathway, glyphosate interferes with the bacteria, algae, fungi, and plants' ability to biosynthesize vitamins, hormones, and amino acids.[38]

If you read through the patent, which is available online, it seems highly likely that ingesting crops sprayed with glyphosate would impact the microbiota of the human digestive tract, through this same effect. If it works as an antibacterial, then it should function as an antibacterial when you ingest it, even if you are *using* it as an herbicide. Given glyphosate's widespread use, it may well be having a profound impact on the microbiomes of many systems and species, starting with soil microorganisms, and moving all the way up the food chain to the microorganisms in our own guts.

This may partly explain why Dr. Theirry Vrain has found an extremely strong correlation between the increase in glyphosate use and the increase in incidence of many diseases that are associated with deficiencies in gut bacteria—such as autism (R = 0.99), diabetes (R = 0.97), obesity (R = 0.96), and dementia (R = 0.99).

---

38 US Patent number 7771736 B2, "Glyphosate Formulations and Their Use for the Inhibition of 5-Enolpyruvylshikimate-3-Phosphate Synthase."

He explains his theories in his lecture "Engineered Food and Your Health: The Nutritional Status of GMOs."[39] Other researchers have shown that glyphosate increases rates of cancer, birth defects, kidney disease, and other health problems.[40]

Welcoming Back the Wild Messiness of Life

So what can we do about the fact that our modern health-care system and modern food processing systems have been on a rampage to wipe out our inner companions? Pharmaceutical researchers are already jumping in to fill the void. But instead of telling patients to breastfeed, have more skin-to-skin contact, avoid industrially grown foods, and eat more raw and lacto-fermented foods, these private laboratories are now patenting and genetically engineering "beneficial" bacteria.

I'd suggest that, rather than waiting for pharmaceutical companies to sell us partial solutions at enormous costs, we start doing our own work to restore our collective microbiome. After all, the collective microbiome of humanity represents not only our future herd immunity but also the future of our emotional intelligence.

First we have to make peace with the fact that bacteria and even intestinal worms are not all bad, that clean isn't always the same as healthy, and that sterile doesn't always equate with safe. (Even if you still get squidgy about germs, you have to realize that there are only seven billion of us on the planet, and there are five nonillion—5×10^{30}—bacteria, taking up more biomass than all the plants, humans, and other animals on Earth. Each of those bacteria is able to evolve faster than you can say "antibiotic." Really, it's time to make friends.)

39 Thierry Vrain, "Engineered Food and Your Health: The Nutritional Status of GMOs," https://www.youtube.com/watch?v=yiU3Ndi6itk.
40 Jeff Ritterman, "Will Richmond Reject Monsanto's Roundup? The Case for Banning Glyphosate," http://www.fooddemocracynow.org/blog/2015/feb/24-1.

For years I have taught that we need to honor and restore our inner ecosystems as well as our outer ecosystems in order to be healthy and vibrant now and in the future, and I have proposed that the second wave of medical progress needs to focus on dealing with the *side effects* of the effective removal of germs from our soil, our food, our homes, and our bodies.[41]

We need to welcome in a wide variety of microorganisms, as if they were our prodigal sons and daughters. And we need to welcome, along with them, the complexity and unpredictability of self-organizing communities and the communal mind-set, symbiotic values, and creativity that come with them. Not just on the microbial level, because the campaign of sterility has extended far beyond the surgical theater and canning factories; it has swept through the offices of doctors and psychologists, into our homes, our schools, our lives, our landscapes, and even our hearts.

During the same time period that we took on the goals of conquering bacteria and subduing nature for our own human benefit, we developed a huge amount of fear and anxiety around dirt, sharing, closeness, "wildness," and community living. Doctors started advising mothers to feed their babies "clean" formula from sterilized bottles. Children were put into cribs and away from the warm bodies they were meant to be with, for fear of germs. Nursing homes with professional doctors and nurses were touted as cleaner, safer places for elders than having them live with their families. Housewives started scrubbing furiously with antiseptic products, while teachers taught children to avoid strangers at all costs. Nurses started handing out forms for us to sign promising layers of privacy and secrecy, and psychologists started installing extra doors in their offices so that clients never had to cross paths with each other.

41 As this manuscript was being edited, scientific and popular articles about the microbiome started popping up all over the place. Interestingly, none of them gave credit to natural medicine or traditional cultures for having kept these concepts alive during the 150-year campaign of medical sterilization of our guts and lives. Few, if any, of them mentioned the role that lacto-fermented and raw foods play in keeping those microbiomes biologically diverse and well populated.

Now we are afraid of things that are "complicated" and "messy." We are afraid of relationships themselves, and have forgotten the lessons that our bacterial companions teach us—that life is a wildly complex, collaborative, creative process, from inside to outside, from start to finish—from the inoculation of our digestive tracts with good bacteria in the birth canal to the hard work of the soil microorganisms that help to grow our food and that will someday turn our bodies back into beautiful fertile earth at the ends of our lives.

Like the laboratory doves I took care of in college, many of us now spend our days in artificial surroundings, protected from germs with hand sanitizers, communicating with our friends from a distance, with our creativity expressing itself mostly by our choices of the industrially made foods we eat or reject. Really, though, we were born for something much more interesting.

Walking Through Another Living Being

Increasingly, the Earth around me seems alive.

Like the microorganisms I've been writing about, I see complex relationships nested within other relationships, as well as indivisible manifestations of the whole.

While picking fiddlehead ferns, last year's spores stick to my feet and repopulate the areas I traverse. Cultivation and harvesting become seamlessly integrated with the land, just by my moving through it. Burdock seeds cling to my legs as I stretch for a hard-to-reach berry, and my boys disperse milkweed and dandelion in their roughhousing as we walk through a field to see the line of rocks the beavers are setting in place across the river. These relationships benefit us in future years, as we eat dandelion pancakes and steamed milkweed pods, gather the beavers' sharpened sticks for staking garden plants, and cook up stir-fried burdock and dried wild leeks.

Over time I've learned to know things in pictures and smells and sounds, lessening the need to look things up or write things down. I know where the turkey-tail fungi and chaga will pop from the trees, offering powerful medicine for my cancer patients. I've learned—in a way that I can't forget—that St. John's wort has side effects of sun sensitivity: from seeing the white spots literally peel off of our cows, leaving the black spots intact, when the heifers accidentally browsed in the meadow where St. John's wort grows thickly.

I know the places where the bright-blue indigo milkcap mushrooms and the tiny hedgehog mushrooms with their adorable spikes will spring up each year to add to our bounty. I know the places where the rare black raspberries grow, and how long to wait between black raspberries and wild blackberries.

There is also a sound that I'm aware of in my body (though it is not audible to my everyday ears): a subterranean hum that tells me I belong in this world—a reflection in my own cells of the sound of the whole. It's a symphonic resonance that could only be possible with the accompaniment of trillions of organisms, from microscopic to majestic, busily working, eating, reproducing, learning, growing, resting, dying, and decomposing in and around each other, creating more and more life and complexity.

It sometimes seems to me that this must be the sound of the unfolding of evolution itself: the "is-ness" of an unnameable creative force moving through time. I suspect this might be the same as the inaudible "OM" emitted by Tibetan prayer wheels, the unspeakable "I AM" of the Torah, and whatever it was that led a young Jew to ask his disciples over and over again to "open" their ears that they might hear. Whatever it is, I am in awe of it.

As I walk through this huge living being, I see the history, as well as the future, of medicine and agriculture. The species that surround me are neighbors, with long histories between our families.

"Oh, hello!" I say, as wild lettuce comes into view, towering above my head like a giant, looking down with amusement at the small human who spends hours caring for tiny little lettuce cousins in her garden.

"Aren't you glorious . . . " I say, while admiring the loops and baubles of wild cucumber climbing a dead tree, as if decorating it for an early Christmas, surrounded by the lacy white flowers of wild carrots.

"All right, all right . . . easy now . . ." I say, navigating around the wild parsnip and nettles that could hurt me if I touched their leaves while harvesting them.

I am struck silent when I walk through the prehistoric landscape of straight, leafless horsetail plants along the Ompompanoosuc River, near the old mill site. The plants seem to be like the Earth's antennae for the ancient sound of the universe I've been feeling vibrate within me. The silica in them, which gives them their rigid structure and their medicinal benefits, stretches back to pre-human history, but it also links them to the era we are in right now—a silicon-based era of intense communication and interconnection through computers, allowing us to measure, understand, and show each other the direct impact of the industrial era on the planet. The horsetail quivers as I walk through it, sending signals into the future.

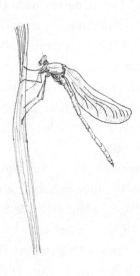

CHAPTER THREE

Medicine, Money, and the Global Pie

I didn't become a health-care provider right away: my body led me there. I graduated from college during the economic boom of the 1980s and got a job working at a major magazine in New York City, deep in the world of capitalism. I shared a ten-by-twelve-foot office in midtown Manhattan with four heavy smokers and a nonsmoking, bespectacled former newspaper writer named Allan, who took me under his wing. Allan had an embarrassing last name, which he said with dignity each time he answered the phone.

Our job was to write, edit, proofread, and fact-check special advertising sections. The department was euphemistically called "Creative Services." Our subjects were Real Estate, which was booming; Vacation Dreams, which we had to imagine; and Sports and Fitness, which was just plain comical. Some of us were thin and some of us were wide, but none of us had ever seen the inside of the gyms we wrote about, and we complained about having to walk a few blocks from the subway to the finish line of the marathon in order to interview runners.

When fact-checking, we got to speak to Donald Trump, Leona Helmsley, Mayor Koch, ambassadors from India and France, and other skyscraper dwellers, while we made $16,000 a year. We wrote about swimming with sea turtles and driving race cars, while we sat in a smoke-filled room with windows that didn't open, cutting text and photos with X-Acto knives, and staring into computer screens with glowing green letters that emitted small but continuous amounts of radiation.

By age twenty-six, my body was a wreck. I developed a cough that wouldn't go away, I had headaches every day, my periods were horrendously painful, my pap smears were abnormal, and my back ached constantly, sending sharp pains down my legs. I went to doctor after doctor, but they didn't have much to offer me, other than pain killers. I was still functional, but by no means was I actually healthy.

Health Care as a Means of Keeping Workers Functional

Although it appears that we are in charge of our own health, many of the choices we make about how to take care of ourselves are based on an underlying motivation, which is built right in to our health-care system: to get back to work as quickly as possible. Everyone is busy trying to keep up with rent or mortgage payments, utility bills, health insurance, student loans, car payments, and credit card payments. So, since people can't afford to actually take time off from work to rest and recover, our health-care system is geared primarily toward keeping people *functional*, which isn't always the same thing as healing or preventing illness.

Here are a few North American cultural assumptions that may be worth examining:

- It's normal to work forty to sixty hours a week, with one to two weeks of vacation per year. Anyone doing less is not contributing his or her share to society.
- Taking care of yourself is not something you should be paid for.
- People who earn more money are entitled to better insurance, better standard and alternative medical care, better nursing homes, and more options for care.
- Being able to work is the measure of our health and worth.
- People who are at a stage of life where they don't work, such as children and elders, are not as "useful" or interesting to talk to as people who have jobs.

- Old people who don't have a lot of money, people with disabilities, people who are trying to process a lot of feelings, and people who have a chronic illness are an emotional and economic drain on families.

Illness, including "mental illness," is considered a social and economic liability in our culture, yet this is ironic, because much of what we consider "illness" is really the body's very clever attempt to heal itself. Fevers burn off viruses. Pain stops us from damaging our joints and muscles with overuse. Crying relieves stress. Fatigue encourages us to rest. Symptoms give us clues that there is an underlying problem that needs to be addressed, and that it is time to pay attention to our bodies and our emotions. Yet we do our best to cover up symptoms and make them go away.

What does our current economic and medical system do to keep people functional? It anesthetizes pain, lowers fevers, removes gallbladders, uses hormones to stop annoying hot flashes, and prescribes drugs to make people wake up, sit still, cheer up, and calm down. These treatments address the symptoms and allow the person to get back to being "functional" but rarely address the underlying cause. This is *reactive* medicine, rather than responsive or preventive medicine.

Not everyone agrees that health and functionality are the same thing. The World Health Organization, for example, defines health as "a state of complete physical, mental, and social well-being and not merely the absence of disease or infirmity."

During my five-year stint in the smoke-filled office without windows, I was unwilling to simply take drugs to subdue my symptoms.

Luckily, I was dating a carpenter named Tony who had a graduate degree in medical anthropology. Hearing me complain nonstop for the first month we were dating, he suggested that I go to the Integral Yoga Institute and try a class.

In those days, yoga was very fringy and mysterious. I loved the dark, quiet rooms. I loved the sacred chanting at the beginnings and endings of classes. I loved the white outfits the teachers wore, and being asked to notice the feeling of my body relaxing into the floor. I loved the way the person at the front desk spoke warmly and respectfully to me while handing me a towel, and I loved the way my symptoms started melting away as I got stronger, more limber, and more hopeful about life.

On Wednesday evenings after work, I began studying ancient Indian texts in the yoga teachers' training program with Swami Asokananda—an American monk with a long beard who wore saffron high-tops to match his robes (and who also showed me how to jump over stadium partitions to get better seats at baseball games). I learned, among other things, that the word *yoga* is from the same root as the word *yoke*—to bring together, to connect. It is similar to *ligio,* the root of the words *ligament* and *religion.* Religion (*re-ligio*), I realized, was meant to reconnect, or relink, things that have broken off from the whole. This felt like what I was experiencing in my own body. Suddenly my undergraduate degree in "Oriental Studies" started to seem as if it might actually be useful. Soon I was teaching yoga on the side, after work, and thinking about how this concept of reconnecting related to my own life and health.

As my health steadily improved, I decided to explore alternative medicine as a career. I spent the next winter studying with an experienced acupuncturist named Robbee Fian, who was practicing illegally, half-hoping to get caught, as she had a lawsuit prepared to argue for the legalization of acupuncture in New York State.[1] Five of us crowded into her small apartment and learned shiatsu, a

---

1   Acupuncture was legalized in New York State a year later in 1992 and Fian went on to become the president of the American Association of Acupuncture and Oriental Medicine.

traditional Japanese form of bodywork using pressure and heat on the same pathways used by acupuncturists. I loved working directly with my hands on people's bodies—and I noticed that my own life-long problem with cold hands had disappeared.

In 1991 Rupert Murdoch sold our magazine to a new conglomerate corporation, and I was given a choice: I could take on two people's jobs for the same meager salary, or I could be laid off (thus saving a coworker her job) and collect unemployment. It was perfect timing.

I sent off two applications: one to a four-year program in acupuncture and herbal medicine in Seattle, the other to a massage school so I could get licensed in shiatsu and help to pay my way through school.

As I collected my things from the office, a young coworker in the art department named Heidi poked her head in the door and said, "When you finish acupuncture school, you should move to Vermont. Trust me. You will fit right in."

Profiting from Illness

Artist Steve Lambert is traveling around the US with a sign saying "Capitalism Works for Me," and asking citizens to vote "True" or "False."[2] What interests Steve is not just the vote coming out of this, but also the conversations he is having with people as they think about how to vote. One conversation with a physician caught Steve's attention: "Capitalism is working for me," said the doctor, "but it's not working for my patients." The doctor went on to say that most of the illness he sees is caused by capitalism.

---

2 Justin Ritchie, "Episode #36 Art into Action" interview with Steve Lambert, The Extraenvironmentalist, podcast audio, February 16, 2012, http://www. extraenvironmentalist.com/2012/02/16/episode-36-art-action/ and personal correspondence with Steve Lambert.

What does he mean? What is the relationship between capitalism, health, and health care? And maybe more importantly: what is the relationship between the growth economy (the need to make greater and greater profits because of the foundation of debt that our economy is based on) and our desire to look out for each other's well-being?

The doctor that Steve interviewed, a specialist in endoscopic surgeries, explains that innovation in the medical profession is driven by investment, which allows people to invent new products and new technology. On the one hand, he sees that innovation is a good thing, because we have more tools with which to diagnose and treat illness, but on the other hand, when you put it all together, there is something very dark about the whole setup. Innovation is only needed, he says, because we *let* people get unhealthy, and that is the unsettling reason for why we are at the forefront of technological advancements. He says capitalism works for *him* as a doctor for one reason only: because if the system was supporting everyone to do what they are supposed to be doing—taking good care of themselves, eating well, spending time with their families, and having a meditative practice—he'd be out of a job.

The White House Asks for Our Opinions

Just after Barack Obama was elected in 2008, the Obama–Biden transition team called for small meetings around the country to discuss problems with the current health-care system, and I was invited to one of those meetings. I had been practicing alternative medicine for fifteen years, and this was the first time I had ever been invited into a meeting with mainstream providers.

First, we were asked to make a list of all the problems we could think of with the current health-care system. One of my neighbors, an oncology nurse, took notes on a large piece of paper, while the health-care providers around me called out their ideas:

- "Doctors don't have enough time to spend with patients."
- "Uninsured people go to the emergency room for basic care."
- "High prices for insurance, and high medical costs for the uninsured."
- "Doctors are stressed out, and overworked, which leads to more medical errors."
- "No one in the medical profession feels fulfilled with their work, because they can't practice in the meaningful way they want to."
- "There is no funding for preventive care."
- "Insurance companies refuse to pay for certain things; preexisting condition clauses."
- "Bills get sent back and forth with nitpicking details. Different rules for each company."
- "Providers' offices are overwhelmed with insurance paperwork, creating higher costs."
- "Doctors can't afford to work on their own because of high malpractice insurance rates."
- "There is no funding for research on drugs that aren't expected to sell well."
- "We pay more for medicines and procedures here than in other countries."

The proposed meeting agenda from the White House then asked us to rank a list of possible solutions they had come up with for the health-care crisis (which included a three-tiered "public" option that perpetuated the inequities of our three-tiered economic and class system). But none of the options the White House was offering seemed to address the root of the problems we had listed.

The people in my group were not exactly my peers—alternative providers got little respect from standard providers in those days—

but I took a deep breath, and asked those gathered to turn the topic of the meeting toward the idea of a total rethinking of our medical system. The room became quiet.

I posed a hypothesis: is it possible that profit is the root of all the big troubles of our current system? If everyone working in health care, including those developing drugs and technology, were paid a decent wage, but no one was making a profit, would the big problems go away?

People nodded. They seemed interested in what I was saying, so I continued. I suggested that most of the problems we see in both standard and alternative health care today, and even in people's *health* today, are related in some way to the way profit motives influence health care, and that our health would improve dramatically if we removed profit from every aspect of health care.

To my surprise, the doctors, nurses, psychologists, and medical researchers at the meeting were open to my idea, and they started giving examples from their own life and work of times when money had completely trumped ethics in medicine. Many of their examples were shocking to me, and two in particular stood out because they demonstrated the way profits influenced even nonprofit organizations.

In the first example, a doctor saw architectural plans for a new renovation at a so-called nonprofit university-based hospital, alongside a map of the current hospital. As he looked at the plans, he realized with horror that the little numbers drawn on each area were not square feet, but rather dollar amounts. Each area was mapped out based on the income it currently provided, or, in the case of the renovation, the income it was expected to provide. The new space was designed to maximize revenues, with less space for such areas as drug detoxification, which tend to bring in less money, and more space for high-profit activities, such as heart surgery. People's actual health needs didn't seem to be reflected in the design at all. For example, the new hospital's design disregarded the fact that the area's local population desperately needed more inpatient rooms for people trying to recover from addictions.

Another example offered at the meeting was from someone who had worked on research projects that were funded by pharmaceutical companies but housed in "nonprofit" universities. The researchers were routinely asked to sign "gag rules," which stated that if they leaked any information about the research results without permission from the pharmaceutical company, they could lose their jobs. This meant that even if research was showing something dangerous about a drug that was about to hit the market, no one could talk about it without permission from the company funding the research.

Nonprofit hospitals and university research labs are supposed to deliver services for the public good, which the government would be delivering if nonprofits didn't exist. They are allowed to be nonprofits because they are acting as a proxy for the government itself. Yet according to Paul Starr, Pulitzer Prize–winning author of *The Social Transformation of American Medicine*, nonprofit hospitals are often a "beehive of corporate activity," and include many profit-making activities that don't affect their tax-exempt status.[3]

In medicine, the two worlds of for-profit and nonprofit are often inextricably intertwined, both ethically and financially. And how could they not be? Although many hospitals, universities, and insurance companies qualify for tax breaks as nonprofits, they still operate entirely within a profit-based medical economy. It seemed clear to me, from my own experiences and the stories I was hearing, that something needed to shift, not just in my own life, but also in the larger health-care system.

---

3   Paul Starr, *The Social Transformation of American Medicine: The Rise of a Sovereign Profession and the Making of a Vast Industry* (New York: Harper Collins, Basic Books, 1982).

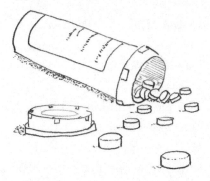

Creating Illness: The Power of Advertising

My friend Marie worked for many years as the "Director of Care Management" at a small hospital, but this didn't stop her from falling into a health-care advertising trap. During a routine physical, a doctor asked Marie if she had any issues with urination. Marie mentioned that ever since she had given birth to her first child, she had to get up a couple of times a night to pee, and had to stop work to urinate several times a day. The doctor, who was sitting in for Marie's regular doctor, told her that she had symptoms of something called "overactive bladder syndrome" and that there was a new drug she could take called Detrol. Marie filled the prescription and started taking it. The need to get up at night lessened, but she developed strange side effects. She went online to do some research and realized that both she and her doctor had been duped.

In the late stages of a growth economy, the things that are being sold get further and further away from the basic necessities of life. The useful, easy-to-sell items are already being marketed, so people start trying to trick each other into buying things that aren't actually useful. You can see this at work in all aspects of our society— including health care—with more and more products and services (that have less and less to do with our actual needs) being pushed at us with increasingly aggressive advertising.

Author Melody Peterson, in her book *Our Daily Meds: How the Pharmaceutical Companies Transformed Themselves into Slick*

Marketing Machines and Hooked the Nation on Prescription Drugs,
describes how Pharmacia corporation created a fictional illness
called "overactive bladder syndrome" in order to get people to buy
the drug that Marie was given.

Peterson attended a global summit of pharmaceutical marketers
where the vice president of Pharmacia gave a presentation entitled
"Positioning Detrol, Creating a Disease." During his presentation,
the executive explained how the marketing campaign unfolded.
First, long before the public first heard of the drug, the company
paid to have articles about "overactive bladder syndrome" (the
invented illness) published in a prominent medical journal, *Urology*,
so that doctors would already be thinking about it when patients
came in to request the drug.

Then they let the public know about the "epidemic" of overactive
bladder syndrome through the news media, which reported that it
was a "serious affliction affecting as many as one in four adults."
These news reports (prompted by press releases from Pharmacia)
came out weeks before Detrol hit the market.

Next, Pharmacia paid doctors to talk publicly about the
"profound" effects that having to urinate nine or ten times a day
could have on a patient's life—from sexual dysfunction to emotional
problems. Finally, Pharmacia hired the actress Debbie Reynolds
to create a public awareness campaign about "overactive bladder
syndrome" and the treatment that was available with the wonderful
new drug called Detrol. Reynolds gave interviews about it to the
Saturday Evening Post and other media.

Susan Brody picked up the story for the *New York Times* health
column, and soon a new disease was born. But so was a new problem. Detrol has many side effects, including anticholinergic effects
that create Alzheimer's-like symptoms of dementia in some patients
who are taking it, particularly if they are on multiple medications.
Unfortunately, once you have convinced the public that they have
a serious disease, it is harder to convince them not to take the
medicine.

A few months later, my friend Marie was getting recurrent urinary tract infections, and she went back to her original physician. He was able to trace it back to the prescription for Detrol. He suggested that Detrol was causing her to retain urine unnaturally, creating an environment for infections, and that she should go off the drug. "But what will I do about needing to pee too frequently?" she asked.

He laughed, "Marie, you learned that in nursing school, you teach it to patients! All you have to do is retrain your bladder, by waiting a little longer each time, until it is back to a normal schedule. It will take a few weeks, and you'll be fine."

She did as the doctor suggested, and quickly relearned how to sleep through the night and urinate at more reasonable frequencies during her workdays.

Many new diagnoses, including "osteopenia" (low bone density), "premenstrual dysphoric disorder" (irritability before menstruation), "GERD" or "gastroesophageal reflux disease" (heartburn), and "social anxiety disorder" (shyness) are actually relatively benign, commonplace issues that have been relabeled as full-fledged disorders in order to sell drugs.

Vince Parry, a pharmaceutical branding expert, traces this strategy back as far as the 1920s, when the manufacturers of Listerine purposefully created anxiety around a new condition called "halitosis" (bad breath) in order to boost sales of an antibacterial product used topically for things like wound healing. In advertisements, the manufacturers played on people's insecurities: blaming halitosis for everything from lack of career advancement to divorce. In response, sales of Listerine jumped from $100,000 to $4 million over the next six years. In a chilling article in *Medical Marketing and Media*, Parry calls this process "the art of branding a condition," noting that marketers are now taking their ability to create new disorders "to new levels of sophistication"[4]:

---

4   Vince Parry, "The Art of Branding a Condition," *Medical Marketing & Media*, May 2003, 43.

Today, the seeds must be sown in a complex landscape of audiences involving pharmaceutical companies, external thought leaders, support groups, and consumers; and the effort must be coordinated with multiple communications agencies in the fields of branding, advertising, education, and public relations.

If done appropriately, condition branding has numerous benefits, the greatest of which is how it creates consensus internally and externally. Such consensus serves to keep brand managers and the clinical community focused on a single story with a lock-and-key problem/solution structure.[5]

Pharmaceutical manufacturers, on average, spend $19 on advertising for every $1 spent on research.[6] That's because it is much easier and more profitable to develop new customers than to develop truly useful new drugs.

The Case Against Competition in Medicine

Even if you think competition is a useful creative force in other economic areas, it's important to understand that in health care, competition and the quest for profits do *not* actually increase quality *or* keep prices down. The whole concept of a "competitive market" assumes that there are consumers shopping around for high quality and good deals. But in medicine, consumers do not actually have access to the information they would need in order to shop around.

During my financial crunch, I went to get a mammogram. I walked into the hospital for my appointment and was sent down the hall to the registration desk. While there, I explained to the older woman behind the desk that I wanted to know ahead of time how much it

5   Ibid.
6   Donald W. Light and Joel R. Lexchin, "Pharmaceutical Research and Development: What Do We Get for All That Money?" *BMJ*:345, August 2012.

would cost. Since I had a $10,000 deductible for my health insurance, I knew I would end up paying for the mammogram out of pocket.

"The last time I got a simple blood test at the hospital down the street it cost me $700, and I still haven't paid it off, so now I always ask first," I told them.

As soon as I said that, the woman handed me a clipboard and a pen. "You need to sign this form before you can get your mammogram," she said.

I looked it over. Basically the form said that I promised to pay for all bills, and all legal fees associated with nonpayment of bills.

"But I can't sign this form until I know what the charge is going to be!"

She looked tired of me—and she had only just met me. She rolled her eyes and said, "This is going to be complicated." She called across the room to a woman from billing.

"How much will the charge be for a mammogram?" she said to her coworker, with a tone clearly meant to prove to me that my question was pointless.

"I don't know," said the woman from billing, without looking up from her desk.

"See?" said the older woman, "we don't really know."

"How can we find out?" I asked, undaunted.

They both went down the hall to ask someone else, leaving me to read the "patient's bill of rights" on the wall.

Time passed.

"We don't have that information," was the answer that came back.

"Well, *someone* here must know!" It seemed absurd to me that the people in billing couldn't find out a price.

"Let me check something." The woman from billing went and got a procedure code and read it to the woman who was checking me in, who then tried to decipher the list of charges.

"Look, it says here that it's $250 for the mammogram, but there's no way for us to know how much the radiologists who read it charge, because they bill separately."

"Right. We don't know that part," agreed the coworker.

"Can we find that out?" I asked.

"I think it's about $35," said the woman from billing, cheerfully trying to settle this conversation.

I persisted. "That's fine, but I'd like to know for sure."

She and I walked down the hall to the radiology department. Luckily the hospital was not very busy. I seemed to be their only patient.

A young, confident-looking woman with jet-black hair at the desk in radiology started looking around in her computer and said, "Well, the mammogram itself is $125 . . . now let's see what the radiology charges are."

"No, the mammogram is $250, we just looked it up," said the billing woman.

"Oh, I'm sure it's less than that," said the younger woman, with a confidence that was no longer reassuring, "but the reading by the radiologists . . . hmmm . . . I don't know. I *think* it's about . . . $175?"

In the end, *no one*—not in billing, nor in the specific departments themselves—could tell me the full price of the mammogram. They all agreed that they just didn't know; they didn't have access to that information.

I went back to the woman at registration and said I was sorry, I couldn't sign the form. So she canceled my mammogram, and suggested, as I was leaving, that I cancel my insurance as well.

"Really, why?" I asked.

There was something in her tone and facial expression that had shifted. I could tell she had decided she liked me, and I found myself trusting whatever she was about to say.

"If you were uninsured, we would charge you very little for this mammogram, or any other procedure. But since you do have insurance, even though you have a $10,000 deductible, we will have to charge you at whatever the highest rate is—that's something I know for sure. And around here, if you are uninsured, you'll actually get better care."

I went home and canceled my health insurance.

I was lucky. After a long and somewhat scary waiting period, in which I was literally relying on the kindness of strangers for my health care, I became eligible for inexpensive health insurance through the State of Vermont.

A Supermarket Without Prices

What would it be like to shop at a supermarket without price tags, and then be told at the checkout counter not to worry—someone will bill you later? What if the cashier asked you, as you loaded your items onto the counter, to sign a form saying that you were responsible for the bill, and for any legal fees that arose if, after you received the bill, you couldn't afford to pay it? What if you were told that the prices actually varied from person to person—not based on their income, but based on negotiations the market made with other, third-party participants? Who would shop at a supermarket like that?

Yet this is exactly what we face as consumers in the world of medicine. Very few people know how much medical treatments cost, nor is it possible to find out in a time frame that would allow patients or providers to compare options. Prices for health care— even if they are known—aren't stable or predictable. The market is segmented, and transactions are hidden. Therefore, you *can't* shop around because there is no easy way to do a price check. This is the first reason that health care in the US is not a "free market" or "competitive market" in the usual sense of those words.

The second reason that health care is not a competitive market has to do with the fact that insurance companies operate as middlemen between patients, caregivers, and the institutions of care, so people don't *have* to think about prices. This leads to a situation in which both consumers *and* providers in the United States act like some teenagers do when they have access to a parent's credit card: not caring how much something costs, or whether it is the best value; simply racking up one charge after another. No one takes full responsibility for evaluating the costs or considering the effects of their spending on the steadily rising prices.

In a single-payer system like Canada's, national insurance pays for *all* the heart medicine that is prescribed to Canadians, so they can negotiate a set price with the manufacturer that applies to everyone in Canada. This gives the Canadian government market power to keep the cost of drugs relatively low and stable, which is why drugs cost less in Canada than in the US. Here, different insurance companies and hospitals are willing to pay widely varying amounts for the same medication or procedure because no one knows what anyone else is paying, and patients who are insured are made to feel as if they are paying nothing at all, which of course is not true.

Even with Medicare, federal law prohibits the US government from using its buying power to negotiate lower prices with pharmaceutical companies—which, if it were allowed, could save the government an estimated $1.4 billion a year.[7]

The cost of even simple drugs varies wildly depending on the place and setting, with some hospitals routinely charging $1.25 for a single aspirin—that's *100 times* the price a patient would pay at a drug store. A nutritional supplement called L-Glutamine, which I sell at my clinic for $37, costs $300 at the Walmart pharmacy. For an opiate such as Percocet, it might be the other way around, costing far more on the street than when doled out by a pharmacist.

The Difficulty in Calculating Value

Knowing what things are worth in health care is also intrinsically more confusing than in other markets.

With automobiles, people know what they are getting and what they are spending. You know that a Ferrari goes faster than a Ford, and that it will also cost more to repair. If you buy a used car, you can look it up in a book or online and see what it is worth. If a new

7   Ethan Rome, "Big Pharma Pockets $711 Billion in Profits by Robbing Seniors, Taxpayers," *Huffington Post*, April 8, 2013.

car doesn't work the way you expect it to, you have a warranty. Not so in medicine.

How, exactly, does one assess the comparative value of a drug or procedure in which there are no guarantees of outcome? Is Prozac a better antidepressant than Wellbutrin? Is surgery to remove a tumor better than radiation to shrink it? The same procedure could save one person's life but end another's, while having no effect whatsoever on someone else. So how do you calculate its value? Doctors have a hard time helping patients navigate choices in health care because the system is too complicated and there is simply too much to know, so price does not operate as a signal of actual value and outcome. Therefore the free market fails in its *information* role in health care in a way that is quite different from other markets.

The most common argument for keeping health care in the private (profit-making) sector is that the quest for profits creates a competitive market and by having a competitive market, the quality of health care goes up while costs go down. Advocates of this free-market approach argue that having a free market, where customers can shop around, improves the quality of health care because people pay more for things that are better. But it simply does not work this way. We have been participants in a great test of this theory, and it turns out that it isn't true.

The United States spends far more on health care than other countries do—nearly double that of the rest of the "developed" world—and the quality and outcomes are dramatically *worse*.

The Institute of Medicine ranks US citizens' health and life expectancy at the bottom of the seventeen most developed countries in the world, while we spend more of our GDP (17.9 percent) and more per capita than the other sixteen countries.[8] Compared to all other countries, the World Health Organization ranked the

8   Steven H. Woolf and Laudan Aron, editors, *US Health in International Perspective: Shorter Lives, Poorer Health* (Washington, DC: National Academies Press, 2013).

US health-care system thirty-seventh in the world—when looking at life expectancy, quality and speed of services, privacy, and fair distribution of services.[9]

Do Investors Understand Medicine?

So if competitive markets aren't creating better-quality health care, then where does the "capitalist" or investor belong in health care? There's no doubt that people who take care of other people, develop drugs, perform surgeries, and figure out puzzling scientific questions should be paid well. These are fine jobs, which often require years of education and experience to do well. These are jobs that change people's lives and save people's lives. Yet the "capitalist" is rarely the researcher, the surgeon, the nurse, or the biochemist. The capitalist hires these people, and makes money from what they do.

Nowadays the capitalist or investor is usually a group of people: CEOs and stockholders. Most of them don't necessarily need to know anything about medicine—other than about the potential profits to be made. Do investors really have our health as a priority?

Let's say we pay the doctors and researchers their salaries, the same as ever, so they will have just as much motivation to keep working on cures. If the costs were shared by the people who participate in the system, why would we need the stockholders siphoning off billions of dollars for their own pockets?

Perhaps even more importantly, why should there be people making *decisions* in our health-care system whose main objective is to make a profit? How does this influence the treatments we are offered, and the ones that are left off the list? On an even larger scale, how has capitalism itself—and the competitive mentality it is based on—changed our view of what the terms *health* and *health care* mean?

---

9   The World Health Report 2000: Health Systems: Improving Performance," World Health Organization, accessed May 27, 2015, www.who.int/whr/2000/en/.

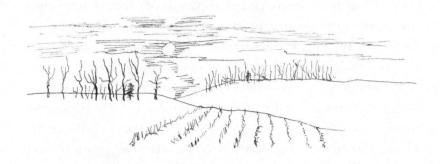

Why People Are Always
Trying to Sell Us Stuff

"The growth economy is not sustainable, because it needs more
of everything to exploit into infinity . . . If you keep creating more money forever, debt expands forever, and the need to
create goods and services expands forever. But we are running
out of nature that we can turn into goods, and we are running
out of community that we can turn into services. So we have
what is now being referred to as 'Peak Everything.'"

—Charles Eisenstein[10]

When profit, rather than necessity, drives innovation, the things
being sold tend to get further and further away from basic human
needs, and the real needs are often forgotten in the rush toward
novelty. No one pointed that out to me more clearly than Charles
Eisenstein.

A friend emailed me a link to a video of Eisenstein, with a note
saying, "I think you should marry this guy. He's like a male version
of you."

Eisenstein had also started off as an alternative medicine provider,
went through a period of financial instability, and started writing

10 Charles Eisenstein, Lecture, Goddard College, February 2012.

books about how larger systems at play in our society have interfered with our ability to care for each other. I jumped in my car the very next week to attend his lecture on economics. (I didn't marry him, but I was impressed by his way of explaining things.).

The reason society is so full of unnecessary costs and everyone is in more and more debt, Eisenstein explained, is because all money is created in the form of *interest-bearing* debt by the Federal Reserve. There is no gold, and there are often no actual bills printed. Each time a bank gets money from the Federal Reserve to loan out to its customers, it is simply creating more debt at the center, and passing it along to the next borrowers.

The growth economy *needs* to keep growing because the entire economy is based on an ever-growing debt. To pay back that ever-increasing debt, borrowers have to find more and more things to sell, and more and more people to sell them to. Profits need to keep increasing.

So how do you do that? Eisenstein noted: "If you try to sell water to people who have perfectly good water to drink, there isn't much money in that, but if you take away the rights to access clean water and then sell bottled water to people, there is a lot of money in that. If you say 'I'd like to empower people to heal themselves,' there isn't much money in that. But if you disempower people from healing themselves by creating lots of rules and regulations about who can practice, and then offer them healing, there is a lot of money in that."

Both Democrats and Republicans are still tied to the idea that if all businesses and investments keep *growing*, people's standard of living will increase as they get more and more stuff, higher-tech health care, and bigger houses to live in with more fun things in them. Everyone will get richer, happier, and more comfortable year after year.

Unfortunately that isn't true. Once people's basic needs are met, having more and more things doesn't actually make us happier.[11]

---

11 Bill McKibben, "Why Having More No Longer Makes Us Happy," *Alternet*, March 21, 2007.

"Because there is always more debt than money, the system is set up to throw us into competition with each other," says Eisenstein. "Scarcity, anxiety, and competition are built right in to the system."

The money-making strategies we tend to come up with in a growth economy are often linked to extraction of natural and social resources, to be doled out to the highest bidder, rather than to the creation and regeneration of common resources, to be shared with all. Because of this, the whole concept of the growth economy may actually be detrimental to our health and to our long-term survival.

In 1972, while I was a fourth grader counting beans at my alternative elementary school in Cambridge, Massachusetts, Donella ("Dana") and Dennis Meadows were sitting in their offices at MIT, just down the street, stuffing punch cards into mammoth computers. They were trying to figure out what would happen if we continued to have unchecked economic and population growth in a world with finite resources.

They wrote about the results in a now-famous book called *The Limits to Growth*. The computer modeling showed that if we did nothing to intervene, we would overshoot the Earth's capacity to support us, and end up in an environmental and social crisis midway through the twenty-first century—essentially a collapse of the modern social and economic system that we have become used to.

But they weren't the first people to point this out. In 1776, Adam Smith, considered by many to be the father of capitalism, warned that economic growth could not continue forever because population growth would push wages down, and natural resources would become increasingly scarce.[12]

---

12 Adam Smith, *An Inquiry into the Nature and Causes of the Wealth of Nations* (Chicago: University of Chicago Press, 1977).

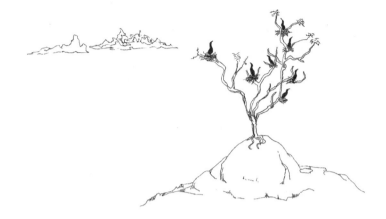

Our Personal Slice of the Global Pie

"Nature uses as little as possible of anything."

–Johann Kepler

Behind every object we use, there is a land-based story. Each window in our home, each toothbrush we buy, each bottle of Tylenol we open, each pair of underpants we put on has an autobiography that involves the use of bioproductive land somewhere else in the world. Some forms of land use are regenerative and create more resources; for example, certain types of farming and ranching practices actually improve the fertility of the soil, create cleaner water, and improve habitat for other species. Most of our current interactions with land, however, are *extractive*—meaning we use up resources faster than the Earth can regenerate them. Petroleum, old-growth forests, and prairie soils are examples of resources that we have used in an extractive way.

If you think of the Earth's resources as a pie, there are three reasons we have been overshooting our planet's capacity since the 1970s:

- Consumption—We buy a lot more stuff (clothes, shoes, cars, computers) than people used to. *Our appetites are getting larger.*

- Population—It's getting crowded at this table, so we have to share the Earth's resources with a lot more people than we used to. *The slices of the pie are getting smaller.*
- Biocapacity—There are fewer natural resources for us to share each year, because we are using them in an extractive way rather than a regenerative way. For example, we are cutting down old-growth forests faster than they can regrow. *The pie itself is getting smaller.*

When I first met Jim Merkel in 2005, he was giving a slide show about Kerala, India, at a local nightclub in Vermont. He was wearing old green rubber boots that went up to his knees; he reminded me of a gawky teenager showing off his science project. His book *Radical Simplicity: Small Footprints on a Finite Earth* had just come out, and he was selling it on a sliding scale from zero to infinity.

Not too long before that, Jim had been working as a top-secret military engineer involved in the arms trade. Deeply troubled by the US invasion of Iraq and by the Exxon *Valdez* oil spill, he left his job and decided to try living in a way that used only what he calculated to be his fair share of the Earth's resources. Having grown up in a large working-class family with a truck driver for a dad, Jim was used to sharing things.

In *Radical Simplicity,* Merkel points out that in order for the world to actually support us, resource-wise, and keep everyone in a state of health and well-being, we each get a certain piece of the pie. The amount we use is called our "ecological footprint."[13]

The Global Footprint network estimates that we would need another half of an Earth to keep supplying us with what we are currently using in the way we are using it. Now consider that the population on Earth has tripled in my mother's lifetime and doubled in my own. Based on estimates from the United Nations,

13 The ecological footprint concept and calculation method was developed as the PhD dissertation of Mathis Wackernagel at the University of British Columbia in Vancouver, Canada, from 1990 to 1994.

if we don't learn how to regenerate what we are using we will need two Earths to supply our appetites by 2030.

Politicians often hold up our current US living standards as a model of what everyone in the world should have—a reason to promote democracy, capitalism, and growth economies around the world. Yet in an extractive economy, we are entirely dependent on other people's (and other species') resources to live the way we do. If everyone lived like an average resident of the US, a total of four Earths would be required to regenerate humanity's annual demand on nature.[14,15]

What does this have to do with health, and health care? In an extractive economy, each dollar we spend represents resources—topsoil, clean water, fish, trees—that take time to be replenished, and without which we cannot be healthy. If we continue with our extractive economy, in order to live within our actual ecological means we each, like Jim Merkel, would have to limit our ecological footprint to match that of people in countries where an annual income of $2,000 to $5,000 is enough to live on. That's $2,000 to $5,000 per year for *everything*: food, transportation, housing, heat, clothing, entertainment, electricity, water, taxes (for things like town maintenance of your road, interstate highways, and wars that your country chooses to engage in), education, and health care itself. *Yet people living in the United States spend an average of $9,523 per person per year on health care alone.*[16]

Part of the reason the US health-care system is so expensive, and so ineffective, is that much of the system is not actually geared toward creating health. Instead, it is geared toward creating wealth:

---

14 Global Footprint Network, http://www.footprintnetwork.org.

15 World Wildlife Foundation, "Human Demand Outstrips Global Supply," http://wwf.panda.org/about_our_earth/all_publications/living_planet_report/2012_lpr/demands_on_our_planet/.

16 US total expenditures were $9,523 per person in 2014. "National Health Expenditures 2014 Highlights," Centers for Medicare and Medicaid, http://www.cms.gov/Research-Statistics-Data-and-Systems/Statistics-Trends-and-Reports/NationalHealthExpendData/Downloads/highlights.pdf.

to make a profit and keep money flowing toward shareholders. Most of the money never reaches the people who are doing the work of caring for others; rather, the main beneficiaries are the people and institutions that invest in an ever-more-complicated health-care infrastructure—the result of the strange collision of the growth economy, high-tech industries, and the human body.

Why Is Our Health-Care System So Expensive?
My retired doctor friend Dale Gephart called me up on my birthday with an unexpected gift. "Have you seen the IOM report? It's exactly what you've been trying to explain to people about the unsustainability of our current system," he said.

On September 6, 2012, the highly respected Institute of Medicine came out with a consensus report in which they examined the state of the US health-care system. As I opened it up and read it, I was filled with both relief and sadness. Finally the medical system was taking its own pulse, but the consequences of having avoided a checkup for so many years were even more shocking than I had expected. The report showed that the United States health-care industry wastes an estimated $750 billion a year on unnecessary services, repeated tests, paperwork, fraud, and missed prevention opportunities, while failing to deliver reliable, top-notch care.[17] This waste is roughly equivalent to the annual budget of the Department of Defense, or the 2008 bank bailout.[18] In addition to this huge amount of waste, we suffer an estimated 75,000 unnecessary deaths per year.[19] That's really sad for people in the United States, but it's even sadder for the rest of the world.

17 Mark Smith, et al., eds., *Best Care at Lower Cost: The Path to Continuously Learning Health Care in America* (Washington, DC: Institute of Medicine of the National Academies, 2012).
18 Annie Lowry, "Study of US Health Care System Finds Both Waste and Opportunity to Improve," *New York Times*, September 11, 2012.
19 Mark Smith, et al., eds., *Best Care at Lower Cost: The Path to Continuously Learning Health Care in America* (Washington, DC: Institute of Medicine of the National Academies, 2012).

What Americans waste on unnecessary health care are resources that other people rely on just to survive.

In 2011, authors N. D. van Egmond and B. J. M. de Vries wrote that the global crisis predicted by Donella and Dennis Meadows would not show up in one clear and visible way: *"Instead, it will appear as a slow erosion of the capability to manage adequately an ever more complex and interdependent reality. It will take the form of a manifold of ecological, financial-economic and social crises."*[20]

My colleague Dan Bednarz points out that this is *already* happening and can be seen if you look at the whole picture: the recent housing crisis, the hurricanes, decreasing clean water supplies, and the steadily rising prices of food and health care. Yet because it doesn't show up in one obvious way, we don't notice that it's happening—even though it is starting to affect us every day. Health care is like the canary in the coal mine: it's one of the more obvious places we can see it, but because we don't understand that it is part of the bigger problem, we call it a "health-care crisis" instead of "a clear example of the limits of the growth economy."

Working Class Acupuncture

During the financial crisis of 2008, while I was struggling with my own debts, my patients were also struggling to afford visits with me. I felt an increasingly difficult tension between the need to increase my own income and the desire to treat people for free or reduced rates. It seemed like an impossible situation—somebody, or maybe everybody, was going to lose. But I ended up figuring out a way to provide my patients with more treatment for less money, and to get

---

20 N. D. Van Egmond and H. J. M. de Vries, "Sustainability: The Search for the Integral Worldview," *Futures* 43 (2011):853–67. (Similar processes are described by Jared Diamond in *Collapse: How Societies Choose to Fail or Succeed*.)

myself out of debt at the same time. It also created more supportive relationships within my whole community. It was based on a regenerative rather than extractive economic model.

Alternative medicine has not been immune to issues with money. Slick advertisements for acupuncture often show a wealthy-looking blonde woman swaddled in sterile white towels receiving her acupuncture facial in a private room, complete with exotic bamboo leaves and flute music.

Not covered by most insurance companies, and costing $50 to $150 per treatment, getting acupuncture once a week costs between $200 and $600 per month, out of pocket (and once a week is often not frequent enough to bring results). At those rates, only a fraction of the population can afford acupuncture. So practitioners are also competing with each other to attract that wealthiest fraction of the population to their practice.

This high-priced model of acupuncture is not necessarily a reflection of the practitioners' social awareness: rather, it reflects the assumption of competition we've all become accustomed to by operating in a profit-based health-care system in general. When health-care providers need to compete for patients, there is an incentive to hoard information and dole it out carefully to the highest bidders—i.e., patients who have the financial resources to pay top dollar for private sessions. It's part of the extractive economy. That's the model I was trained in.

Then I attended a workshop given by a group from Portland, Oregon, called "Working Class Acupuncture." They were advocating a new business model that was the polar opposite of the high-cost "spa model" of acupuncture. At their own clinic, Lisa Rohleder and Skip Van Meter, cofounders of the Community Acupuncture movement, treated patients in a group setting for a fraction of the cost of a usual treatment and ended up with a thriving business.

When I first met her, Rohleder was explaining to a group of acupuncturists that practitioners working in the "spa model" have always tried to market to the sensibilities and desires of wealthier patients who can afford high rates, rather than attempting to create a practice that is accessible to the general public. Rohleder pointed out that wealthy patients pay those high prices mostly for privacy, for a feeling of specialness, being "fussed over," and one-on-one attention, which are highly valued commodities among wealthy people[21] but completely unnecessary for acupuncture to be effective.

Rohleder explained that working-class people, on the other hand, tend to value simplicity, practicality, sharing resources, group activities, and the kinds of strong bonds that form during tough times. Having straddled both sides of the class divide for much of my life, I immediately understood what she was getting at, and I was intrigued. I thought back to the camaraderie of the friendships I had formed while working as a waitress in a dingy pizza joint in Michigan, and how I was still in touch with those women, years later, while there were people in the wealthier branches of my family who seemed too caught up in their investments to notice that I still existed. I imagined the Rockefellers in my practice getting treated alongside the friendly guys who worked in the town garage, and I thought there might be some benefit to everyone to try a group treatment setting.

A Low-Cost Model of Care, Without the Need for Fund-raising

When she was starting her own practice, Rohleder looked around at other clinics and saw that at current prices, acupuncture would never be affordable to her working-class family and friends, so she decided to do something different. She set up a group treatment space (in what had been an old cement-floored TV repair shop), scheduled treatment slots every ten minutes, and set the clinic's rates

---

21 I can say from having treated some of the wealthiest people in the world that these values come from childhoods that are often a strange combination of privilege and neglect.

on a no-questions-asked sliding scale of $15 to $35—essentially splitting the cost of a private visit, and passing the savings along to those who wanted to join in the fun.[22] In came construction workers, hotel maids, motorcycle repair people, elderly Jamaican women, social workers, and late-night waitresses, all lounging in beach chairs together in a funky inner-city loft, getting treated for PTSD, asbestos inhalation, cancer, digestive paralysis, and more. Rohleder and Van Meter decided to call their clinic "Working Class Acupuncture."

This community acupuncture model, now practiced by hundreds of acupuncturists around the world, is one of the most socially equitable treatment models out there, and it completely bypasses the health insurance industry and all the paperwork associated with it. After a quick check-in, the needles are inserted and the patient relaxes and often goes to sleep for thirty to ninety minutes. During this time, several more treatments can be started while the acupuncturist keeps an eye on everyone else.

Intrigued, I decided to incorporate inexpensive group treatments into my schedule. I was tired by the end of each day, and sometimes it felt like I was working as a waitress again as I moved from table to table, but it felt good to work hard, and I was able to help many more people. In the past, when I was charging higher rates, people would often give up after three or four treatments, even if they were slowly improving, because they simply could not afford to keep coming. Now they could come for eight, twelve, or twenty-four treatments and actually solve the problem that brought them to my clinic.

Watching my acupuncture successes double and triple as more people were able to afford regular weekly treatments for longer stretches of time, I started thinking more about socially and economically resilient medicine. This new way of working highlighted how

22   Lisa Rohleder, L.Ac., *The Remedy: Integrating Acupuncture into American Health Care* (Portland: Kulia Waiwaiole, 2011).

the values of the wealthy had created the sterile, aloof, airbrushed image of what health care was "supposed" to look like, and how different it could be—and might *have* to be—if the economic crisis hit any harder.

In the community model of care, the intention is to set the sliding scale low enough that anyone can afford to come for treatment—which, in turn, expands the potential client base from just a fraction of the population to nearly everyone. Patients don't need to "qualify" by proving they are poor, or feel guilty about using the services if they are rich. The acupuncturists who work in community acupuncture clinics end up making about the same amount per hour as they would in a "spa model" clinic, but they have a much more stable income, and less worry about competition. Unlike other low-cost clinics, which are dependent on federal aid or private grants, there is no fund-raising or grant writing to be done. Therefore, Rohleder points out, community acupuncture is not charity work; it is a very useful business model with widespread social benefits.

Social Benefits of Group Treatments

The benefits of group treatment are not just economic. Primates are social creatures; we evolved to feel comfortable hanging out in groups. Perhaps because of this, group settings have clear health benefits,[23] and like many others who have shifted to this model I've noticed that there is something that happens in a group setting that is quite different from what happens in a private room. Rohleder and Van Meter write:

> Treating patients in a community space . . . allows a unique kind of synergy to kick in. When everyone in the room is in a state of deep relaxation, the energy of

---

23 Julianne Holt-Lunstad, et al., "Social Relationships and Mortality Risk: A Meta-analytic Review," *PLoS Med* 7, no. 7 (2010), accessed June 9, 2015, doi:10.1371/journal.pmed.1000316.

each individual treatment spills over into the whole and creates a powerful shared state, similar to the experience of group meditation—even though the majority of our patients are not meditators. That shared state in turn makes each of the individual treatments more potent. From that perspective, the community model allows us to do more for each individual, for less money.[24]

Acupuncturists working in this model don't necessarily feel that they are working harder, even though they are seeing three to six times more patients in a day. That's because the group dynamic has a supportive quality in and of itself, which puts less pressure on the acupuncturist to give everyone special attention.

The patients are creating the healing atmosphere as much as the practitioners are, which helps all of us remember where the real strength resides . . . One acupuncturist commented that she thought that what was most useful about this model is that it de-emphasized everyone's ego. The setting makes it clear that nobody is more important than anybody else is, and the acupuncturists are facilitating something rather than *doing something to* the patients. It helps patients not to focus too much on their individual problems and to remember that, no matter what is going wrong for them personally, we're still all in this together.[25]

This is an example of a regenerative economy: not using up social resources, but creating more.

24 Lisa Rohleder and Skip Van Meter, *Working Class Acupuncture for Patients* (brochure), 22.
25 Ibid.

Cooperative, Rather than Competitive, Businesses

As their own success became clearer, Rohleder and Van Meter kept encouraging other acupuncturists in Portland to try their model, and an interesting thing happened: the more clinics that opened, the busier all of them got. Rohleder attributes this to a number of factors:

- When people can come more often, they get better faster.
- When a treatment strategy is inexpensive and works well, people tend to talk about it.
- When everyone can afford to get treatment, the only limit to the business model is the population density of the area.

In other words, the net result of having multiple clinics in Portland has been more and more pain-free, relaxed people walking around, telling other people how great and affordable acupuncture is compared to other types of health care. Not to mention, there are more satisfied acupuncturists making a living doing something they love.

Since then, the model has spread around the US and the world. Community acupuncturists, in turn, have joined together to set up a multi-stakeholder cooperative called the People's Organization of Community Acupuncture (POCA). POCA's mission is to "make acupuncture available and accessible to as many people as possible and to support those providing acupuncture to create stable and sustainable businesses and jobs."[26]

Multi-stakeholder cooperatives recognize that producers and consumers are mutually dependent, and that the health of the relationship between these groups is connected to the health of the larger community and economy. Members of POCA, therefore, are

26 "POCA's Mission," People's Organization of Community Acupuncture, accessed September 20, 2012, https://www.pocacoop.com/our-mission-and-vision.

a mix of acupuncturists, patients, and even prospective patients who want to bring a clinic to their town, each of whom receives a wide range of member benefits, including mentorship and microloans for starting clinics in underserved areas. In 2012, POCA's membership included approximately 500 acupuncturists, 500 patients, 250 clinics, and 5 other organizations.

In the thirty-five-minute film *Community Acupuncture, the Calmest Revolution Ever Staged,*[27] acupuncturists talk about the problems of having an "acupuncture mortgage"—student loan debt of up to $100,000—from attending acupuncture school, which is now a four-year program requiring a BA and many pre-med courses. This sort of debt has kept many acupuncturists from considering working in low-income or rural areas, and has kept other qualified people from even considering a career in acupuncture.

POCA's answer to these two concerns has been to create a unique and affordable acupuncture school, "POCA Tech," which opened in 2014, specifically for training new acupuncturists who are planning to work in community acupuncture clinics in underserved areas. The curriculum reflects POCA's values of social justice and removing hierarchy from the health-care world. The tuition—$5,800 per year—is a fraction of the cost of most acupuncture training programs.

Why Isn't Community Acupuncture a Basic Part of Our Health-Care System?

In 2003, the World Health Organization (WHO) published "Acupuncture: Review and Analysis of Controlled Clinical Trials."[28] The WHO analyzed research results up to 1998 and came up with a list of nearly 100 illnesses for which acupuncture was an effective treatment. Many more years' worth of positive research has accu-

---

27 Ibid.
28 World Health Organization, "Acupuncture: Review and Analysis of Reports on Controlled Clinical Trials," Accessed September 20, 2012, http://www.who.int/iris/handle/10665/42414#sthash.NM45uTCb.dpuf.

mulated since this document was first published. Acupuncture is starting to show itself as a very viable treatment for hundreds of disorders—everything from infertility to back pain.

If community acupuncture can safely be used to provide treatment for so many disorders for as little as $15 per session, with no side effects and very little environmental waste, why would a health-care system insist on more expensive, more dangerous, and less environmentally sound treatments? (And why bother with insurance coverage?) As the social, economic, and environmental costs of medicine rise, acupuncture is one of the first places communities should look for help in providing effective, affordable care. The community acupuncture model is helping this transition to happen in a way that can benefit the entire population while bypassing the need to wait for legislative or insurance reforms.

The Gift Economy

When an accountant first heard about my sliding scale, she was dumbfounded that I allowed people to decide for themselves how much they wanted to pay. "Why would anyone pay more if you give them a choice? If you went to Walmart and the item had a price tag of $25 to $50, everyone would pay $25!" I told her that my patients routinely paid all up and down the scale, and sometimes even insisted on paying higher than the top of the scale, because they know me and how hard I work, and because they know that their money helps to support a more equitable local economy, and a healthier group of neighbors. This is an example of what is called a "gift economy."

As for me, I have excused myself from the debt-based economy. By buying only the things I actually have the money to pay for, I find myself living a more realistic, and ultimately more satisfying, life. Using this strategy, over a five-year period I was able to stabilize my income and expenses, help far more people afford my treatments, and pay off $70,000 of credit card bills. I ended up free of unsecured debt.

My clinic is not fancy, and it is sometimes embarrassingly chaotic as it intersects with the new economic limits of my life—no money to build closets or buy a dishwasher—but unlike many other businesses in the area, mine has become more and more solvent. By using this new community-supported health-care model, I have survived an economic roller coaster.

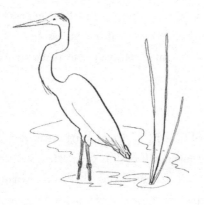

CHAPTER FOUR

Who Defines "Normal"?
Rediscovering Our Inner Compass

"If medicated means complacent, it helps no one . . . When we are overmedicated, our emotions become synthetic. For personal growth, for a satisfying marriage and for a more peaceful world, what we need is more empathy, compassion, receptivity, emotionality and vulnerability, not less."

—Julie Holland, psychiatrist[1]

Partly because of pharmaceutical marketing tactics, the reported incidence of "mental illness" is escalating wildly.

In 1950, many adults had lived through World Wars I and II and the Great Depression, and were facing the looming threat of nuclear war with the Soviet Union, so it is a little surprising that only one in 10,000 adults were thought to have depression. This incidence was so low that when the first antidepressant was made that year, there was little interest in marketing the drug.[2] But by 2005, after a slate of new antidepressants had exploded onto the market, researchers estimated that one in five adults had had a depression-related mood disorder at some point in their lives.[3] This is over a *two-thousand-fold* increase. In his article "The Art

1   Julie Holland, "Medicating Women's Feelings," *New York Times,* March 1, 2015.
2   Melody Peterson, *Our Daily Meds: How the Pharmaceutical Companies Transformed Themselves into Slick Marketing Machines and Hooked the Nation on Prescription Drugs* (New York: Farrar, Strauss, and Giroux, 2008).
3   Lifetime Prevalence Estimates, http://www.hcp.med.harvard.edu/ncs/ftpdir/ NCS-R_Lifetime_Prevalence_Estimates.pdf.

of Branding a Condition" (written for a medical marketing magazine), Vince Parry notes, "No therapeutic category is more accepting of condition branding than the field of anxiety and depression, where illness is rarely based on measurable physical symptoms, and is therefore open to conceptual definition."[4]

After the pharmaceutical company GlaxoSmithKline hired a public relations firm to market Paxil for shyness in 1999, the appearance of the phrase "social anxiety" in the press rose from about fifty to more than 1 billion mentions in just two years. Shyness—in the guise of "social anxiety disorder"—became the third-most-common "mental illness" in the US. Meanwhile, the advertising campaign for Paxil as a drug for shyness picked up an award for the "best campaign in the United States."[5,6]

One out of four women in the United States is currently on some sort of psychiatric medication. Abilify, an antipsychotic, is the number one best-selling drug in the United States—among *all* medications, not just among psychiatric medications.[7]

The DSM (*Diagnostic and Statistical Manual of Mental Disorders*), published by the American Psychiatric Association, is used by doctors, psychiatric nurse practitioners, licensed social workers, insurance companies, and pharmaceutical companies to look up the symptoms and suggested pharmaceutical treatment of mental illnesses. The manual has expanded from 106 mental disorders in 1952 to more than 300 disorders in 2013. Many of these so-called mental disorders are things that were never considered disorders until there were drugs available to treat them. Consider these:

4   Vince Parry, "The Art of Branding a Condition," *Medical Marketing & Media*, May 2003, 46.
5   Carl Elliott, "How to Brand a Disease—And Sell a Cure," CNN, October 11, 2010.
6   Ray Moynihan, "Selling Sickness: The Pharmaceutical Industry and Disease Mongering," *BMJ* 324 (2002).
7   Julie Holland, "Medicating Women's Feelings," *New York Times,* February 28, 2015.

- *"Premenstrual Dysphoric Disorder"* (marked irritability or anger, mood swings, interpersonal conflicts, or food cravings the week before menses starts)
- *"Female Sexual Interest/Arousal Disorder"* (including reduced interest in sexual activity, reduced erotic fantasies, reduced initiation of sexual activity, and typically unreceptive to a partner's attempts to initiate sexual activity)
- *"Male Hypoactive Sexual Desire Disorder"* (deficient sexual/erotic thoughts or fantasies and desire for sexual activity for a minimum of six months)

Parry, writing to an audience of pharmaceutical marketers, notes, "Not surprisingly, many of these newly coined conditions were brought to light through direct funding by pharmaceutical companies, in research, in publicity, or in both."[8]

Fewer and fewer of us are considered normal, and more and more of us qualify to be medicated. But who is defining "normal"?

Of the 170 DSM panel members responsible for developing and modifying the diagnostic criteria for mental illness, a recent study showed that more than half of them had one or more financial associations with companies in the pharmaceutical industry. Every one of the members of the panels on psychotic disorders and mood disorders (such as depression, bipolar, seasonal affective disorder, postpartum depression) had financial ties to pharmaceutical companies. The authors of the study write, "The connections are especially strong in those diagnostic areas where drugs are the first line of treatment for mental disorders."[9]

Why doesn't the Food and Drug Administration (FDA) step in? Isn't their job to make sure that companies are not pulling the wool over our eyes and selling us dangerous or useless drugs?

8   Vince Parry, "The Art of Branding a Condition," *Medical Marketing & Media*, May 2003, 46.
9   Lisa Cosgrove, et al., "Financial Ties Between DSM-IV Panel Members and the Pharmaceutical Industry," *Psychotherapy and Psychosomatics* 75 (2006):154–60.

USA Today reported that 54 percent of the time, experts hired to advise the FDA on the safety and effectiveness of medicines had direct financial interest in the drugs they were evaluating. Some of these advisors had helped a pharmaceutical company develop a medicine and then served on an FDA advisory committee that judged the drug. Federal law generally prohibits the FDA from using experts with financial conflicts of interest, but *USA Today* found that the FDA waived the restrictions more than 800 times in the two years between 1998 and 2000.[10]

USA Today analyzed potential financial conflicts at 159 FDA advisory committee meetings and found that:

- At 92 percent of the meetings, at least one member had a financial conflict of interest.
- At 55 percent of meetings, half or more of the FDA advisors had conflicts of interest.
- At meetings where broader issues were discussed, 92 percent of the members had conflicts of interest.
- At meetings dealing with the fate of a specific drug, 33 percent of the experts had a financial conflict.[11]

And at the time of the analysis, according to FDA guidelines a committee member could actually be paid up to $50,000 a year by a drug company without any financial conflict being disclosed as long as the work was on a topic other than what the committee was evaluating.[12]

---

10 Dennis Cauchon, "FDA Advisors Tied to Industry," *USA Today*, September 25, 2000.
11 Ibid.
12 Anthony Colpo, *The Great Cholesterol Con* (Lulu.com, 2006), 118.

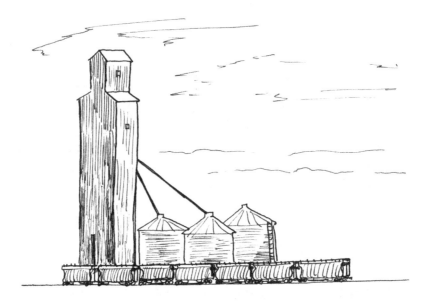

Farmer Brains vs. Hunter-Gatherer Brains

"Knowledge without love will not stick. But if love comes first, knowledge is sure to follow."

—John Burroughs

Each time I hear about another child at our local school who has been put on Ritalin, I cringe. In my own practice I address "attention disorders" by giving patients dietary and lifestyle suggestions and by prescribing a lot of connection to the natural world. But mostly I help to re-frame the issue in broader social and anthropological terms.

Mental "disorders" are largely defined by the cultural and social values that surround us. In the 1800s, Southern doctors used the term "Drapetomania" to describe the mental illness afflicting black slaves who desired to escape to freedom,[13] and homosexuality was

---

13 Arthur L. Caplan, et al., *Health, Disease, and Illness: Concepts in Medicine* (Washington, DC: Georgetown University Press, 2004).

considered a mental illness by the American Psychiatric Association until 1973.

Likewise, Attention Deficit Disorder may well be one of those terms that reveals more about our sedentary, repetitive school culture than it says about the children who are being labeled and medicated.

In 2012, twenty times more children were on addictive, amphetamine-based drugs for attention disorders than thirty years before, and a full 11 percent of children ages four to seventeen had received a diagnosis of ADHD.[14] Drugs like Ritalin and Adderall are often prescribed during an office visit with the suggestion to "see if it helps with focus," as if response to the drug was a diagnostic criterion. The drugs do typically help with the kind of focus needed for repetitive tasks for a time—but that would be true of any stimulant (like coffee), for almost anyone trying it for the first time. The benefits of stimulants soon wear off, though, leaving only side effects and an addiction to the drugs. If children go off the drugs and feel worse, the same odd logic is used: this, parents are told, is an indicator that the children *need* the drugs, rather than being a normal symptom of withdrawal from a stimulant.[15]

People who are diagnosed with ADD and ADHD have brains that are hard-wired to search for new and interesting things. We scan the horizon looking for patterns (yes, me too!), we zoom in on details that stand out or don't fit. We often perform well when there is a crisis going on, but slack off when things are more calm, and start hunting for interesting snacks in the cupboard instead. We tend to be systems thinkers (seeing not just the elephant, but the whole herd) and we can come up with solutions that are outside the box. It's not that we curious and energetic types don't have the ability to pay attention, because with certain activities that involve a lot of novelty—like starting new companies, making art, or hunting

14 L. Allan Sroufe, "Ritalin Gone Wrong," *New York Times Sunday Review*, January 28, 2012.
15 Ibid.

for edible mushrooms—we can go into hyper-focus mode for hours, days, or weeks. The issue is, we get bored easily with certain types of repetitive activities, like washing dishes, memorizing multiplication tables, or sitting in classrooms. Being in school, to people like us, feels like being a hunter-gatherer stuck in a farmer's life.

Recent neuroscience research shows that the genetic variation associated with people who are diagnosed with "attention disorders" (in our agriculturally based society) actually correlates strongly with the genetic makeup and lifestyles of hunter-gatherers. The same genetic variation occurs more frequently in nomadic populations,[16] and it works to your advantage, health-wise, if you happen to be born into a nomadic tribe.[17] Not so if you are born into an agricultural society with our more scheduled, linear, indoor culture.

Meanwhile, drugs such as Ritalin create long-term changes in the brain similar to, and sometimes greater than, the effects of cocaine use,[18] creating more sensitivity to stressful circumstances, increased anxiety, more tendency toward depression, and large increases in "learned helplessness."[19] Giving curious, energetic, innovative children drugs that create learned helplessness is exactly the opposite of what we should be doing, particularly as we enter an era in which interesting and innovative solutions will be essential and we will all need to pitch in. (Interestingly, the single most dependable predictor of adults who are likely to be involved in caring for their environment is how much time they spent in "wild" play outdoors as children.[20])

16 C. S. Chen, et al., "Population Migration and the Variation of Dopamine D4 Receptor (DRD4) Allele Frequencies Around the Globe," *Evolution and Human Behavior* 20, no. 5 (1999):309–24.

17 Dan T. A. Eisenberg, et al., "Dopamine Receptor Genetic Polymorphisms and Body Composition in Undernourished Pastoralists: An Exploration of Nutrition Indices Among Nomadic and Recently Settled Ariaal Men of Northern Kenya," *BMC Evolutionary Biology* 173, no. 8 (2008).

18 "Ritalin May Cause Changes in the Brain's Reward Areas," Rockefeller University Newswire, February 4, 2009, http://newswire.rockefeller.edu/2009/02/04/ ritalin-may-cause-changes-in-the-brains-rewards-areas/?output=pdf.

19 "Ritalin Use in Childhood May Increase Depression," *Harvard Gazette*, December 8, 2003.

20 David Sobel, "Look, Don't Touch," *Orion*, July 2, 2012.

As any drug dealer knows, addictions create long-term customers, and drug companies in a for-profit system are uniquely poised to take advantage of that. With these sorts of changes to the brain, many of the children on Ritalin and Adderall will likely become lifelong consumers of psychiatric drugs and indentured servants to the pharmaceutical companies—creating guaranteed profits for decades to come.

In just four years, between 1991 and 1995, the number of two- to four-year-olds taking stimulants rose by *300 percent*.[21] In 2007, thirty-five times more children qualified for disability benefits because of "mental illness" than twenty years earlier.[22] In 2010, National Institutes of Health data showed that one in five 13–18-year-olds had had a "seriously debilitating mental illness"[23] while nearly *half* of that group had had some sort of mental disorder in their life so far.[24] *What?!?!* Half of all teenagers in the United States have already been mentally ill sometime in their life? Wait a minute . . .

The trend toward medicating children has also created at least one generation of children who think that emotions and behaviors can and should be with treated with pills, leaving them susceptible to addictions, and with strange opinions about their own normalcy.

A Choice . . .

It is time for a radical change of approach. We now know that gut bacteria and blood sugar levels influence mood, and that diets

21 Julie Magno Zito, et al., "Trends in the Prescribing of Psychotropic Medications to Preschoolers," *JAMA* 283, no. 8 (2000).

22 Marcia Angell, "The Epidemic of Mental Illness: Why?" *New York Review of Books*, June 23, 2011.

23 "Any Disorder Among Children," National Institute of Mental Health, accessed September 20, 2012, http://www.nimh.nih.gov/health/statistics/prevalence/any-disorder-among-children.shtml.

24 K. R. Merikangas, et al., "Lifetime Prevalence of Mental Disorders in U.S. Adolescents: Results from the National Comorbidity Survey Replication—Adolescent Supplement (NCS-A)," *Journal of the American Academy of Child and Adolescent Psychiatry* 49, no. 10 (2010):980–89.

that stabilize blood sugar metabolism, and reset and replenish the microbiome,[25] can influence brain chemistry and moods. Mindfulness exercises, regular physical exercise, and contact with nature can help do the same. Perhaps the most important factor in the creation of emotional resiliency is the availability of close, warm, loving attention from other human beings—people who understand how the social context for defining "normal" can influence our perceptions of ourselves and others.

Through many years of treating patients, I have come to believe that as long as the brain's basic structure is intact, "mental illness" can be prevented and treated with a combination of non-pharmaceutical strategies. Our society hasn't yet figured out how to have enough social and economic resources available to *implement* those strategies for everyone, partly because most people haven't witnessed what is possible when nutrient-dense diet, mindfulness, exercise, a relationship with the natural world, and a truly supportive community are combined. (When non-pharmaceutical strategies for mental health are studied at all, they are usually studied in isolation.) Therefore, in the absence of realizing that there are other options, the increasing use of drugs and diagnoses may seem like a reasonable choice.

But I have already witnessed, in profound ways—in my practice, in my own close-knit community of support, and at the elementary school where I work—what is possible when ample social resources are available and multiple strategies for emotional resiliency are combined. If we choose to, we can create the social structures and support systems that will allow all young people to become emotionally resilient and all adults to heal from past hurts.

25 Depending on the situation, I recommend the G.A.P.S. ("Gut and Psychology Syndrome") diet, a ketogenic diet, or some version of a "paleo" diet for patients wanting to work on mood and concentration issues, as well many physiological problems.

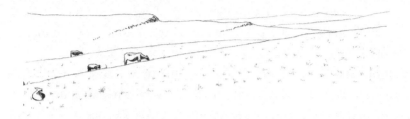

Biophilia

My two sons and I are floating around a bend of the Ompompanoosuc River on our backs, arms outstretched, holding hands. Our bodies are completely relaxed, letting the river hold us. We watch the trees go by above our heads. With our ears just under the water, the only sound we hear is our own breathing.

As we get out and lie down in the sun, we remember the time we saw half of a wild bird's egg floating by around the same bend, like a funny little boat, and how we swam out to catch it and marveled at the little bird embryo inside, taking its only ride down the river. Today, a duck comes honk-honking down the fly-way just a few feet over our heads, zooming around the curves of the river, very much alive.

In winter we return to this same bend in the river and laugh at the odd boinging sound of rocks as we skim them across the ice, trying to hit our targets: the large shards of ice that cracked upwards on a warm day and are now frozen in place.

Each day, we go somewhere so we can see what is really happening in the world.

I learned this love of nature from my parents.

Even though we grew up in the city, my mother made a point of bringing us, and the children in her inner-city nursery schools, out into the natural world whenever possible. When that wasn't an option, she brought other living things inside.

In her classrooms, there were tadpoles turning into frogs and chicks hatching out of eggs. At home there were iguanas hiding in our houseplants, and aquariums full of turtles my mother had rescued from the road. My brother and I spent hours making mazes out of bricks for our guinea pigs and pet rats, and scared our friends with our snakes and tarantulas. Our Christmas tree was decorated with eggs whose insides we had carefully blown out, painted by family and friends, and angels we made of pine cones, with acorn heads and feather wings.

When we lived in Mexico, my stepfather took us out into wilder territory, rafting down rivers surrounded by strange birds, and camping on riverbanks covered with thousands of tiny frogs.

On weekends we stayed with our father and stepmother at their old farmhouse in New Hampshire with no toilet, just an outhouse, and no bathtub, just a nearby lake and a bar of soap. There, my stepmother taught me to grow and can vegetables, make blueberry jam, and embroider. I rode horses at a nearby farm, had a pet chicken, and rolled around on the ground with thirteen puppies biting, scratching, and wrestling with me as one of their own.

It turns out my parents were right to take my brother and me to the country every chance they got, and to bring nature inside when we were in the city.

Hundreds of studies show that spending time in nature and with other species has profound physiological and psychological influences on our health.[26,27,28] The term "biophilia" was originally coined by the psychologist Erich Fromm as a way of describing a particular psychological orientation to all that is alive and vital. Biologist and Pulitzer Prize winner E. O. Wilson—an entomologist who spent much of his life following ants in the jungle—

---

26 "Improving Health and Wellness through Access to Nature," American Public Health Association, https://www.apha.org/policies-and-advocacy/public-health-policy-statements/policy-database/2014/07/08/09/18/improving-health-and-wellness-through-access-to-nature.

27 Howard Frumkin and Richard Louv, "Conserving Land; Preserving Human Health," Land Trust Alliance Special Anniversary Report, 2007.

28 R. S. Ulrich, "Biophilia, Biophobia, and Natural Landscapes," in *The Biophilia Hypothesis* (Washington, DC: Island Press, 1993).

went further and proposed that our subconscious urge to affiliate with other forms of life, and the connections we seek with plants and animals, are rooted in our biology. Wilson defines biophilia as "the innate tendency to focus on life and lifelike processes." He writes, "From infancy we concentrate happily on ourselves and other organisms. We learn to distinguish life from the inanimate and move toward it like moths to a porch light."

Contact with nature can tip the balance toward health and recovery, even if that contact is simply a room with a view. Postsurgical patients who are given a hospital room looking out at a grove of trees recover a full day sooner, and with less need for pain medication, than those whose window looks out at a wall.[29] Prison inmates whose cell windows look out over farmland have fewer illnesses than those whose cell windows look out over a concrete courtyard.[30] Children with a room with a view of nature are more protected from stress,[31] and workers with a view of nature from their office windows report significantly less frustration and more work enthusiasm than those without.

Being out in nature is even better.

Our Inner Compasses
Patients with Alzheimer's who are allowed to go out into a garden at different times of day and experience different light levels show decreased agitation, less wandering, and improved ability to interact in groups.[32] Perhaps this is because the ability to orient oneself—to the sense of place, time of day, and year—through their own

29 R. S. Ulrich, "View Through a Window May Influence Recovery from Surgery," *Science* 224 (1984):420–21.
30 Keith G. Tidball and Marianne E. Krasny, *Greening in the Red Zone: Disaster, Resilience and Community Greening* (New York: Springer, 2014), 365.
31 Gary W. Evans and Nancy M. Wells, "Housing and Mental Health: A Review of the Evidence and a Methodological and Conceptual Critique," *Journal of Social Issues* 59, no. 3 (2003):475–500.
32 D. Carreon, et al., "The Therapeutic Design of Environments for People with Dementia: A Review of the Empirical Research," *Gerontologist* 40, no. 4 (2000): 397–416.

ancient senses (rather than through abstract modern tools, such as clocks, calendars, and maps) helps to orient their brains in other ways, as well, as it does for all of us when we are allowed to spend time outdoors.

Our tissues, including our brains, contain magnetosomes—small quantities of magnetite that interact with larger magnetic fields, like the Earth's. Other animal species share this trait, and some quite clearly show the effects of it: honeybees and certain bacteria can easily orient themselves to magnets,[33] while birds, foxes, and many other animals also have navigational abilities based partly on their ability to sense the Earth's magnetic fields.[34,35] Given that we still have magnetosomes, it is likely that we have the remnants of those navigational capacities ourselves.

People living in traditional cultures spend much more time in direct physical contact with the Earth's surfaces—on dirt or stone floors indoors, and walking barefoot or in thin leather shoes outdoors—maintaining an electromagnetic connection with the Earth. Work in traditional cultures often has people performing tasks in a natural setting, touching plants, trees, and rocks, picking up on natural cues that enhance their sense of orientation as well as their general health. In contrast, modern culture has us living profoundly insulated lives. Those of us living high-tech modern lives rarely, if ever, touch the earth directly with our bare skin.

Is this a problem? It may be—for electrical reasons. Our cells, our nerves, our hearts, and our brains all use electrical signaling systems, and the natural state of our bodies is to have a slight negative charge, just like the Earth and its bodies of water. But when

33 Joseph Kirschvink, et al., "Magnetite in Human Tissues, A Mechanism for the Biological Effects of Weak ELF Magnetic Fields," *Bioelectromagnetics Supplement* 1 (1992):101–13, http://web.gps.caltech.edu/~jkirschvink/pdfs/KirschvinkBEMS92.pdf.
34 Janice G. Mather and R. Robin Baker, "Magnetic Sense of Direction in Woodmice for Route-Based Navigation," *Nature* 291 (1981):152–155, doi: 10.1038/291152a0.
35 K. Schmidt-Koenig and T. W. Keeton, eds., *Animal Migration, Navigation and Homing* (Berlin: Springer-Verlag, 1978).

we are indoors, surrounded by technology and insulated from the earth, the atmosphere around us develops a slight positive charge, which our bodies pick up and build up over time.

This buildup of positive charge when people are separated from the Earth's natural electromagnetic field is associated with many poor health conditions, especially those related to chronic inflammation, including arthritis, fibromyalgia, cardiovascular disease, and gastrointestinal disorders. One's sense of time and space also tends to be off, leading to trouble sleeping, irritability, and anxiety.[36,37] This is probably why we love to lie on the beach, swim in rivers, walk barefoot on the ground, and sit on big rocks.

As an acupuncturist who works with other people's bodies, and as a writer who spends a lot of time working on computers that give off a large electrical charge, I've found it useful to go barefoot on my walks in spring and fall, and jump into the river whenever I can. Immersing the whole body in natural water, like a river, lake, or ocean, is a quick and thorough way to return the body to its natural charge.

In winter, I sometimes sit and do research in my cellar, reading with my bare feet on the ground, which (though not as pleasant as jumping into a river) works pretty well. If all else fails, I'll grab a friend, and find a hole in the ice that the deer have kept open in a still body of water, and jump in . . . It works beautifully to return me to my senses.

Our Sensory Context

Tonight, Henry and Alden and I walk barefoot, squishing around the Zebedee Headwater wetlands, and watch for the bittern, flying heavily up into a tree, his call a low sound that almost mimics the

36 Robert Becker, *Cross-Currents: The Perils of Electro-pollution, the Promise of Electro-Medicine* (New York: Penguin, 1990).
37 Gaetan Chevalier, et al., "Earthing: Health Implications of Reconnecting the Human Body to the Earth's Surface Electrons," *Journal of Environmental and Public Health*, 2012.

bullfrogs. Alden lies on his belly attempting to catch a frog, which keeps disappearing under a grassy bank covered with wildflowers. The beavers, who have created an ornate wood sculpture museum in a mossy corner, swim back and forth nearby, occasionally whacking the water with their tails.

Why do we long for the river, the woods, the mountains, and the bogs? Something keeps calling us back there, because that is where life is happening, where we can remember who we are and where we belong.

The experience of a sense of awe, most often found in nature (but also in art, music, and spirituality) has a profound impact on our capacity to see ourselves in the context of the whole—and to change our behaviors accordingly. Researchers have found that awe (defined as "an emotional response to perceptually vast stimuli that transcend current frames of reference") leads to more ethical decision making, more generosity, more helping behaviors, and less entitlement.[38]

Just as we need the ecology of our inner microbial companions to help our brains and bodies function and develop properly, we also need the ecology of our outer world.

Our noses, lungs, and brains *need* the millions of imperceptible smells, our ears *need* the sounds of crickets and birds and rain, our eyes *need* the movements and colors of leaves and water and insects, the stars at night, and the changing patterns of clouds moving across an open sky, in order to function properly, to orient us, to fit us correctly into the true context of our world. We need to see and smell and hear and feel ourselves in the midst of our coevolved landscape—interacting with our coevolved companions—to understand and sort out what is important and real and true from what is merely what we've been *told* to want by someone trying to sell us something.

38 Paul K. Piff, et al., "Awe, the Small Self, and Prosocial Behavior," *Journal of Personality and Social Psychology* 108, no. 6 (2015), 883–99.

It's not that basketball games and YouTube videos aren't fun and interesting. But the movies we watch, the cars we drive, the houses we live in, the furniture we sit on, the blogs we read—these are all human-made artifacts that were designed by our own brains. Human life has become almost an entirely self-referential world, yet . . . show us a picture on Instagram or Facebook, and our eyes will track toward whatever is living. No matter how urbanized, addicted, or jaded we become, on some level we still long to see and feel ourselves in the context of the whole.

Indigenous Science

> "Humans are not the center of life, nor is any other single species. Humans are not even central to life. We are a recent, rapidly growing part of an enormous ancient whole."
> —Lynn Margulis[39]

Although the men in my family were involved in some of the most profound experiments in disconnection in the history of the world, the women in my family have managed to hang on to their matrilineal home for six generations. It sits on just a few acres in the center of the Adirondack Mountains—the largest national park in the United States—a place known for its wild beauty. It was there, during summers with my grandmother, that I learned to learn in a very different way.

My brother and I would sit for hours in front of a spider's hole in the ground, seeing how long it would take for it to come out. We paddled up and down lakes in wooden canoes, carrying our lunch in woven wicker pack baskets, memorizing the sound of water dripping off of paddles, and learned to catch fish in streams and make fires in corners of huge rocks. We'd pick wild strawberries from the field, and eat them sitting on a glacial rock the size of an

---

39   Lynn Margulis, *Symbiotic Planet: A New Look at Evolution* (New York: Basic Books, 1999), 120.

elephant, whose every crevice and crack we had memorized and named. Although I am not indigenous to North America, I was fortunate enough to experience a deep connection to place.

Iroquois author Paula Underwood writes of indigenous cultures studying plants, animals, and humans *in context* by a "profound immersion in, and awareness of, the whole circumstance."[40] What does she mean by this?

Research, in the indigenous scientific model, is done within the interior and exterior landscape itself—it is purposefully subjective as well as objective. Gregory Cajete, Tewa author of *Native Science: Natural Laws of Interdependence,* calls this "high-context learning."

This is in direct contrast to the "low-context learning" that Western scientists use for research, conducted in sealed laboratories. Low-context learning separates things out from their environment (like doves, children, and active ingredients of plants) in order to examine them.

An Aboriginal teacher from Australia (referred to in the *Australian Journal of Teacher Education* only as "Cathy") contrasted the two styles of learning in this way:

> Western teaching and learning is very compartmentalized. It's very boxed and it has to fit . . . [but] We don't fit into a box. We're surrounding the box. We're part of the box. We're inside the box. We're all over the box. We're like the air, we're all around . . . White teachers don't see that.[41]

Native science, according to Cajete, is based on intimate relationships, unique to a particular people and place. But what is learned

---

40 Paula Underwood Spencer, "A Native American Worldview: Hawk and Eagle Both Are Singing," *Noetic Sciences Review* 15 (1990).

41 Ninetta Santoro, et al., "Teaching Indigenous Children: Listening to and Learning from Indigenous Teachers," *Australian Journal of Teacher Education* 36, no. 10 (2011).

through those intimate localized relationships—through participation, observation, visualization, and stories—is that each part is also participating in a larger web of relationships.

"This idea of the superorganism, which is the planet Earth, has been held by every Indigenous culture that I can remember ever studying and can be said to be the prime philosophy of native peoples," says Cajete. "It is the understanding that one comes to naturally; if you are a good observer you can begin to see how life-forces interact on the Earth or just in the place in which you live, and you begin to have a sense that there is this greater organism, this great process."[42]

It's not just about observation. In his book, Cajete describes native science as being "thoroughly wrapped in a blanket of metaphor, expressed in story, art, community, dance, song, ritual, music, astronomical knowledge, and technologies such as hunting, fishing, farming, [and] healing." Because of this difference from more rationalist science, Cajete says, rationalistic scientists ("the 'younger brothers' of Native scientists") have difficulty understanding the essence of Native science, which is creative participation with nature.[43]

Creative participation includes a spiritual relationship with the land that Cajete calls "ensoulment"—a deep level of psychological and spiritual involvement with one's surroundings.

In my own life and in my work with patients I have seen how this leads quite naturally to an understanding of how to heal and be healed by *leaning in to relationships*, with plants, places, rituals, and community.

We are all native to somewhere, and we all have the genetic capacity—even if it is rusty from generations of disuse—to build

---

42 Paul Racette, "Indigenous Perspectives in GEOSS: An Interview with Gregory Cajete," *Earthzine magazine*, April 6, 2009.
43 Gregory Cajete, *Native Science: Natural Laws of Interdependence* (Santa Fe: Clear Light Publishers, 2000).

relationships with the land, animals, and people around us, to absorb knowledge from the natural world, and to understand the connections between our own inner weather and the storms, floods, and wildfires that surround us.

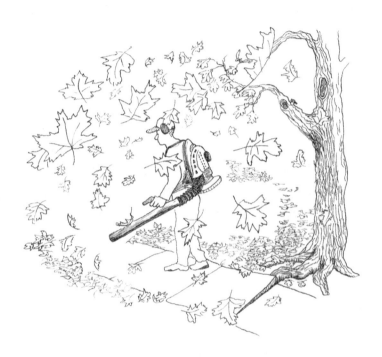

CHAPTER FIVE

Climate, Water, and Health

I generally don't pay much attention to the daily weather predictions, preferring to be surprised, but on a Saturday night in August 2011, when I saw my neighbors at the gas station filling up one container after another for their generators, I knew something was up.

"Hurricanes," said the weather report, *"are great big heat engines, taking warm, moist air and hoisting it aloft tens of thousands of feet into the air. That hot, wet air hits the cold upper atmosphere and makes these clouds. It's basically like smoke from a big chimney, except it's water vapor, not smoke. On the bright side, these types of clouds could treat us to a nice sunset this evening, a small treat that doesn't come close to offsetting what will hit us when Irene roars through."*[1]

When I heard the word "hurricane," I felt myself tremble. Six years before, I had been right smack in the middle of Hurricane Wilma's path during a medical conference in Florida, and the memory hadn't fully left my body. As I tried to translate Florida to Vermont, I was mostly worried about wind—the kind of wind I had had to lean and push my body through, heart pounding, holding hands with colleagues I barely knew, as we climbed down the outdoor staircase from our fourth-floor hotel rooms. The kind of wind that had blown out the upper hotel walls, sent trees flying through the air, and flattened stop signs to the ground, leaving seventy of us stranded for several days in a powerless hotel where we had nothing to eat except canned salad bar items and wedding cakes that were rapidly defrosting in the hotel freezers.

---

1   Matt Sutkoski, "Weather Rapport," *Burlington Free Press*, August 27, 2011.

It started to rain. There were so many trees in Vermont that it seemed hopeless to even start preparing for that kind of wind. I moved anything out of the yard that might fly around and smash a window, and moved my car out from under the tree where it was parked. I filled up some water buckets in case of a power outage, emptied out a small bucket that had started to catch rain from a leak in my roof, and waited.

I got an email from the fire chief asking if I could help out at the Red Cross emergency shelter. I was surprised. I was one of fifteen people in our town who had done a preliminary training several months before, when the elementary school was equipped as a shelter for potential future emergencies. We didn't really expect to ever have to use it. But the chief said that up to thirty families were expected at the shelter that night, and that police and firefighters had been evacuating our neighbors all along the Ompompanoosuc River.

Closing my laptop, I noticed that the bucket had filled up with rainwater, again, even though it seemed like I had just emptied it.

⚓

Later that evening, with Hurricane Irene dumping millions of gallons of rain on our town, I decided I had to see what was going on with my river. A few hours before, I had been appointed shelter manager and I was sitting around with a few other volunteers. Things were fairly quiet. I handed Mike, the owner of the Village Store, the walkie-talkie and told him I'd be right back. It was like checking on a beloved friend. I gathered up my sons from the cafeteria, saying, "Let's go look at the river," and they jumped up and grabbed their coats.

Henry and Alden are well aware of the river's many seasonal, weekly, and daily moods and how they form the liturgical cycle of our year. It's one of the strongest relationships in our lives.

The boys and I ran through the rain to the car, and headed down to the Tucker Hill covered bridge that spans the waterfall that used to power one of many local mills. This was the exciting place to walk out onto the rocks during spring flooding and listen to the roar, to jump in quick and naked while the water was barely moving on a hot summer day, or to sit and watch the water slide over frozen tuffets of ice-covered rocks in the winter.

But we didn't get to the bridge. When we saw that Sharon the dogcatcher's yard was flooded, we stopped and got out. In twenty years I had never seen this happen. How could the water be that high? We started to take a detour on foot, and walked partway down a little path toward the river, but I reached out and stopped Henry and Alden when I saw the river itself. The waves were about eight feet tall as they crested over the rocks—one part was shooting high, high up into the air like a huge rooster comb—while the rest of it went barreling down at a tremendous speed. The bottom of the bridge was not far at all above the torrent of this swollen river.

This bridge had seen some damage over the past decade, with occasional oversize dump trucks ramming through the roof by accident, and a carful of my friends crashing through the wooden wall only to be saved by a doctor who happened to be driving behind them. But as I watched the scene before me, I saw that we could lose the covered bridge entirely today if the water got any higher, or if the Mannings' log yard a quarter mile up the road, which was already starting to fill with water, let loose its stockpiles of hundreds of piled-up trees waiting to be transported and all that came barreling downstream all at once.

I shuddered, and we headed back up to the shelter. I showed Mike and Tig, the other shelter volunteers, the video I had shot on my cell phone and they just shook their heads. They were getting minute-by-minute reports from around the region on the walkie-talkie, which was connected to the emergency and fire departments.

"Bartonsville lost their covered bridge a few minutes ago," said Mike, "and so did Quechee."

In one night of flooding, 200 bridges and 500 miles of roads were washed away just in my small state of Vermont. As we pored over our friends' pictures on Facebook and drove through the landscape over the next week, we saw things we'd never imagined. Cows and chickens and sheep drowned in our neighbor's fields. Well-known stores and restaurants filled with mud and water. Propane tanks washed downriver from a supplier and piled up against a dam downtown. Houses tilted at crazy angles. Roads collapsed, everywhere we went. Community gardens—that we had eaten fresh greens out of just the week before—covered with sewage that had overflowed from the treatment plant.

Our own Ompompanoosuc River had collected a seemingly endless supply of soccer balls, basketballs, and volleyballs, along with trees, plastic bottles, rhododendron bushes, and lawn chairs. But they didn't move, they just sat there on the water, staring at us. The dam was closed to protect towns downstream, and we ended up with a large lake filled with debris rather than a swift-moving river. A Porta-Potty floated on its side, with a bluish cloud of human waste floating on the stagnant water around it. This was a familiar landscape turned unfamiliar.

Stormy Weather

"We are running Genesis backward, de-creating."
—Bill McKibben

Soon after Irene, I heard Bill McKibben speak. Though his home was Vermont, he was out in California, just out of jail for protesting the Keystone XL oil pipeline, and Skyping in to a conference on local resiliency.

Bill, a professor, author, and climate activist, was visibly moved to be talking to his neighbors in Vermont, even from a distance. "How *are* you all?" he said from the screen on the wall, as if talking to family. "How was it? Are you okay??"

People nodded yes, and some wobbled their hands, "so-so."

"Okay, let's talk about this flood, and the two others we had this year," he said.

In a matter of ten minutes, he was able to make it very clear to me what was going on with the climate.

Yes, Bill explained, the world is getting hotter. In fact, that month was the 319th month in a row with global temperatures above twentieth-century averages. In Pakistan, temperatures had reached 129 degrees a couple of years before, and in a variety of places in the world heat waves were killing people.

The issue with "global warming" isn't just about heat, however. The problem with climate change, for much of the world, is actually about how that heat affects the *water* cycle. It's about storms and moisture: places being too wet or too dry.

As more moisture evaporates out of the ground in some places, more moisture is coming down as rain, snow, sleet, and hail in other places. This creates drought and wildfires in some areas, and flooding and mudslides in others. In thickly wooded places like the Northeastern United States, which are near the ocean and already tend to be moist, these shifts can mean dramatically increased rain and flooding.

In Vermont we had three flood emergencies in the 1960s, two in the 1970s, three in the 1980s, ten in the 1990s, ten in the 2000s, and in 2011 we had three major floods in just *one year.*

In dry areas, like much of the rest of the United States, drought is setting in for years at a time. As soil dries out from increased heat and lack of moisture, some types of soil compact into a hard crust, making it even more impenetrable to future rainwater. During heavy rains after a drought, these areas can have drought *and* runoff flooding at the same time. Other types of soils lose their structure entirely and blow away.

Our world is a complex place with an almost infinite number of interconnected natural systems. In complexity, feedback loops can develop that make things better—or worse.

As higher temperatures melt snowcaps on mountains, the mountains are left with bare areas that no longer provide consistent moisture in the area from slow evaporation, no longer cool the surrounding atmosphere by reflecting heat, and no longer provide a slowly melting source of water flowing down into streams and rivers all summer long. This leaves some parts of the globe—like Colorado—with hotter air, higher winds, dried-up vegetation, and dried-up mountain streambeds: the perfect setup for wildfires. When dust from blowing soils settles over snowfields, the snow is darker and absorbs more heat. This compounds the tendency for earlier snowmelt, which feeds back into the rest of the problem.

A Record of Ancient Life Rises to the Sky

I used to think climate change was boring.

But after Hurricane Irene ripped through our town, and after I understood that climate change was about *water*, it became interesting to me. Now I wanted to know about carbon. And the more I learned, the more interested I became.

For a couple of hundred years human civilization has persistently dug, drilled, and pumped ancient carbon out of the Earth: carbon that stores the energy that used to be sunshine, which then became plants (and animals that ate the plants) that slowly compacted into a layer of thick black stuff and explosive gases. Petroleum, coal, and natural gas are all called "fossil fuels" because they come from this carbon-rich fossil layer of the earth and sea.

Years ago, folks said you could poke a stick in the ground in Texas and oil would come shooting out of the earth. That kind of easy oil is all used up.

We made a million plastic doodads out of it: toys for our kids, toys for ourselves, toys for our dogs, and toys for our gerbils. At home we had Tupperware parties, and danced in our polyester clothes made out of petroleum, while listening to music pressed into records and cassettes and eight-track tapes made out of it.

At work, we made pharmaceutical drugs out of the easy carbon chains in it, and soothing salves and ointments with petroleum jelly. We made disposable plastic syringes, pill bottles, and thermometers. We made disposable tubes and disposable IV bags, disposable gloves and disposable bedpans. In hospitals and at home we replaced metal and glass and rubber with it in every way we could think of, so that we could use things once and throw them away and get rid of the germs and not think about them anymore.

We burned it to dispose of hospital waste in incinerators, and we burned it to dig big landfills and to ship garbage out into the ocean where we wouldn't ever have to see it again.

We burned it to heat our homes and our hospitals and factories. We boiled it down to a thick paste and made highways across the globe out of tar, and homes with linoleum floors and vinyl siding and asphalt roofs, and then we burned it some more to drive our cars so we could live far away from work, and vacation even farther away. We burned it to power ships and trains and planes and trucks. We shipped a million plastic doodads around the world, bringing things here from China, and sending stuff back to China. We used up lots of it to build rockets and spaceships and blasted them out into unknown places to see if there were any other planets like ours with water we could drink, and cows walking around that we could eat. (There weren't.)

So we tweaked it in laboratories and created chemicals and weapons in case somebody tried to take our oil, and in-between wars we tweaked those chemicals and made pesticides and herbicides so we could hop on a huge piece of farm machinery and drive around and not have to pull weeds or pick bugs off of our potato plants or talk to our mule when she wouldn't listen. We tweaked it some more and made truckloads full of televisions, telephones, fax machines, computers, printers, and laptops with little plastic keys like the ones I am typing on right now. It was great. It was cheap. It was easy. It was fun.

                                    ✍

When we burn fossil fuels, we vaporize them, via smoke and smog and exhaust, into another form of carbon: CO_2, which is why people talk about "carbon emissions." Much of that CO_2 settles onto the Earth, changing the acidity of the oceans, lakes, and rivers. The rest of it rises up into the atmosphere. Over time, all that vaporizing of ancient carbon has formed a layer around the Earth's atmosphere, similar to the way a cigarette smoker's house has a layer of tar on all the walls.

Each year, that layer of CO_2 we are creating gets denser. It traps more and more heat and doesn't allow it to leave the atmosphere, so the Earth and all its living things have a harder time cooling off. It's like living inside a greenhouse.

For much of human history, the amount of CO_2 in the atmosphere was relatively stable, hovering for 10,000 years at about 275 parts per million. Around the time of the Industrial Revolution, it started rising. In 2012, we were at 392 parts per million and climbing. In May 2013, we had already reached 400 parts per million, and despite the fact that news reporters love round numbers, much of the media was strangely silent.

NASA climate expert James Hansen has stated that anything more than 350 parts per million is not compatible with the climate in which human civilization developed and to which our bodies (and the bodies of most other living things on the planet) are adapted.[2]

2   James Hansen, et al., "Target Atmospheric CO_2: Where Should Humanity Aim?" *Open Atmos. Sci. J.* 2 (2008):217–31.

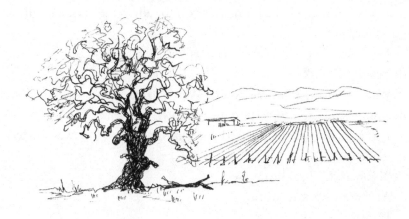

Climate's Effect on Health and Health Care

I called Anna Goldstein, an old college friend of mine, who works at 350.org, the international climate organization started by Bill McKibben and some of his students. I asked her to send me whatever information they had about how climate change was impacting human health and health care.

"I'm just the one who organizes actions," said Anna, "so I'm not the expert you need, but I'll find someone who is."

The next day I got an email that made me feel really weird.

> Dear Didi,
> My name is Meredith and I am a new intern at the 350.org office in Oakland with Anna Goldstein. I am working on a new page for the 350.org website with general information about public health and climate change, as well as what kinds of things people in health-related fields can get involved in. I was told that you are knowledgeable in this area, and I'd love to get your input . . .

I should have felt proud. But when a worldwide organization, dealing with nothing less than the most significant crisis in the history of human civilization, asks you for advice, it's not actually a good feeling.

I was sitting there in my pajamas with a huge pile of unwashed dishes in the sink.

Wait a minute. *I* was the expert? Weren't *real* experts—not people like me—supposed to be doing this stuff?

I stared at my table, covered with messy papers. My eyes started to glaze over.

"Holy shit," I said to myself.

And then I got to work.

I started compiling lists.

Health Hazards of Drought[3]

Drought is a slow and compounding problem and can last for years at a time, having devastating effects on the physical and emotional lives of people in affected regions. Drought reduces the ability to grow and harvest food, whether it is farmed, raised, fished, or hunted, and affects both the quality and quantity of drinking water.

- Drought affects groundwater by *drying up shallow wells* and increasing the *infiltration of salt water* into fresh-water supplies in coastal areas.
- Reduced stream and river flows can *increase the concentration of agricultural and other pollutants in water*. Fish living in these waters *absorb more toxins* and can be harmful to eat.
- Higher water temperatures in lakes and reservoirs lead to *reduced oxygen levels*, which can affect aquatic life and water quality.
- The water that is available has *higher concentrations of toxins and bacteria*, and can develop *algae blooms that are toxic* to animals (and humans) that drink or swim in it.

3 "When Every Drop Counts," Center for Disease Control, accessed June 9, 2015, www.cdc.gov/nceh/ehs/Docs/When_Every_Drop_Counts.pdf.

- Runoff from drought-related wildfires can carry extra sediment, ash, charcoal, and woody debris to surface waters, killing fish and other aquatic life by *decreasing oxygen levels in the water.*
- Filtration systems for clean drinking water easily become *clogged with ash, mud, and other particulates* during drought.
- Crops grown without enough water are *more vulnerable to insects* and certain diseases.
- The plants that grow in poor soil are often of poor quality. Animals fed grain that was grown in poor conditions are *more prone to serious diseases.*
- Dry earth allows more particles to float through the air, which is what happened during the "Dust Bowl" of the 1930s. These particles include viruses, bacteria, and toxic materials that *are inhaled and can create "dust pneumonia" and other illness.*

Health Hazards of Flooding [4,5,6]

While many people rightly fear drowning in a flood, many of the health risks from flooding come after the floodwaters recede:

- *Lack of safe drinking water*—due to contamination of rivers, wells, and reservoirs from debris that has washed into them—can lead to dehydration, diarrhea, and other infections.
- *Toxic mold and mildew infestations,* growing on damp walls after floodwaters recede, can cause severe respiratory

4   Roger Few, et al., "Floods, Health, and Climate Change: A Strategic Review," Tyndall Centre for Climate Change Research, accessed September 27, 2012.
5   Mike Ahern, et al., "Global Health Impact of Floods: Epidemiological Evidence," Epidemiologic Reviews, Johns Hopkins Bloomberg School of Public Health 27 (2005).
6   "Flooding and Communicable Diseases Fact Sheet," World Health Organization, accessed September 27, 2012. http://www.who.int/hac/techguidance/ems/flood_cds/en/index.html.

and allergic problems as people breathe in or come in contact with the spores.

- *Hazardous waste,* such as propane, motor oil, sewage, heavy metals, and chemicals spread throughout the landscape by flooding, can contaminate soil that is used for growing food and outdoor play spaces for children.
- *Increased numbers of insects* that hatch in damp areas— like mosquitoes and ticks—can more readily spread infectious diseases like malaria, dengue fever, and Lyme disease as they feed on humans and animals.
- *A rise in other communicable diseases* from bacteria can occur; in particular, the spirochete leptospirosis can spread as floodwaters wash the infected urine of rodents around.

General Health Effects of Climate Change [7,8,9]

- *Extended power outages* from natural disasters leave people without heat, air conditioning, food, water, and communication, leading to increased *hypothermia and heat exhaustion.*
- People who are evacuated during emergencies often can't get *access to medications* they left behind.
- *Disease-carrying insects* are moving into regions that were once too cold for them to survive, and predators, such as bats, which used to keep them under control, are dying off due to changes in ecosystems.
- More and more people are affected by *acute and post-traumatic stress* from the shock and loss they experience during disasters.

7   Samuel S. Myers and Aaron Bernstein, "The Coming Health Crisis," *The Scientist,* January 1, 2011.
8   "Climate and Health: Diseases Carried by Vectors," Centers for Disease Control, http://www.cdc.gov/climateandhealth/effects/vectorborne_zoonotic.htm
9   "Protecting Health from Climate Change," World Health Organization, http://www.who.int/world-health-day/toolkit/dyk_whd2008_annex1.pdf.

- As clean water and arable land become scarcer, there are *increased conflicts* over these precious resources.
- Increasing numbers of people around the world are *homeless* or *forced to live in refugee camps*, without adequate access to fresh water. This provides an ideal environment for the spread of contagious diseases.

I started extrapolating into the future.

It takes a huge amount of money to recover from each weather event—money that could be going into other things, like health care. The repairs from Vermont's flooding in 2011 cost close to one billion dollars. Many parts of the country and world are already wrestling with huge debt. National, local, and household economies can be stressed to the breaking point when one disaster after another requires money to rebuild and repair roads, houses, businesses, and hospitals. Nationally—and internationally—the number of weather-related events resulting in more than a billion dollars in damages has climbed dramatically over the past thirty years.[10]

Put all this against a background of a rapidly aging and increasingly medicated population, a steady rise in chronic degenerative diseases, an increase in antibiotic-resistant bacteria, and an ongoing financial crisis. Then add to the picture a health-care system that is completely mired in insurance restrictions and paperwork, run by hundreds of large corporations (who do not communicate with each other) trying to manage the very real concerns of the coming era. It's time to start thinking about our whole system, so we can prevent the following:

- Many for-profit health-care corporations and manufacturers of drugs and hospital supplies may close up shop or shift their focus when it gets too hard or too

---

10 "Billion Dollar Weather/Climate Disasters," National Climatic Data Center, accessed September 27, 2012, www.ncdc.noaa.gov/oa/reports/billionz.html.

expensive to make a profit due to uncertain weather and supply-chain problems.

- Nonprofit hospitals, clinics, treatment centers, nursing homes, and public-health agencies may have trouble finding funding as private, state, and federal funds get diverted into disaster relief.
- Care providers may become overwhelmed with changing needs at home and work, including influxes of new patients, power outages, decreased funding, drug shortages, shifting disease patterns, and chaotic weather patterns.

Water, the Basis of Human Health

"Civilization has been a permanent dialogue between human beings and water."

—Paolo Lugari, founder of Gaviotas Ecovillage, Colombia

As I continued researching climate and health, it became clearer and clearer to me that water was not only the key issue with climate, it was the key issue with the future of health care, as well. Building a future in which people, animals, and land could be healthy and resilient would involve addressing the movement and distribution of water—for crops, farms, and people—worldwide.

I came across a government document called "The Intelligence Community Assessment on Global Water Security."[11] It was put together in 2012 by the Central Intelligence Agency, the Defense Intelligence Agency, the National Security Agency, the Department of Homeland Security, the Department of State, the Federal Bureau

---

11 Director of National Intelligence, Intelligence Community Assessment, *Global Water Security*, unclassified version released by the Office of the Director of National Intelligence (2012), http://www.dni.gov/files/documents/Newsroom/Press%20 Releases/ICA_Global%20Water%20Security.pdf.

of Investigation, and the National Counterterrorism Center. Obviously, it is a *very* important document.

Since the US government had been awfully quiet about climate change up until that point, I was struck by the fact that climate change is mentioned multiple times in this document. It lists the Western United States as one area that will "almost certainly suffer a decrease in water resources *due to climate change*," and states that "drinking water from both aquifers and surface water resources almost certainly will further decline in many areas of the developing world, as water quality decreases from *salt-water intrusion* [i.e., rising sea levels and flooding] and industrial, biofuel, agricultural, and sanitation processes." [Italics are mine.]

It goes on: "With one-sixth of the Earth's population relying on meltwater from glaciers and seasonal snowpacks for their water supply, reductions in meltwater *caused by climate-change induced receding glaciers and reduced snowpacks* will have significant impacts."

But here's the scary part. The assessment states that the intelligence community has high confidence in its judgment from multiple reliable sources that *by 2030, humanity's annual global water requirements will exceed current sustainable water supplies by 40 percent.*

Why, I wondered, was the intelligence community so interested in water? This seemed like something that some other part of the government, like the Environmental Protection Agency, should be writing about.

Maria Otero, US Under Secretary for Civilian Security, Democracy, and Human Rights, summed up the answer: "The Intelligence Community Assessment reinforces our view that water is not just a human health issue, not just an economic development or environmental issue, *but also a security issue. We will ensure water issues stay at the top of our foreign policy and national security agenda.*"[12]

12 US Department of State, *Global Water Security: The Intelligence Community Assessment*, last Modified May 9, 2012, http://www.state.gov/j/189598.htm.

Now I was scared on a different level. The CIA, the Defense Intelligence Agency, the NSA, the Department of Homeland Security, the Department of State, the FBI, and the National Counterterrorism Center were thinking about climate change and its impacts on human health and survival far more than they were letting on. But they weren't thinking about how to get solar panels on everyone's roofs. They weren't thinking about funding more public transportation or ending the subsidies to big oil companies. They weren't even thinking about how to get more money into FEMA to pay for all the natural disasters that they knew were going to be happening. No. They were thinking about national security, foreign policy—and maybe even war over water.

I looked at my dog sleeping on the blue linoleum floor next to my feet. I listened to my kids laughing in the next room. I looked at my appointment book full of sixteen patients coming in the next day for help with tennis elbow, anxiety, and allergies to dust mites.

That's when I called Jule. She's part of my circle of peer support—other community leaders I can trade listening time with—so I don't have to settle for feeling depressed and immobilized when I am faced with a fact like the one I was having trouble with at that very moment. Finally she answered.

"Hey."

"I need some help."

"How much time do you want?" Jule asked.

"About ten hours, but I'd settle for fifteen minutes if you have it."

"Okay sweetie, go ahead."

I heard the beep of her pushing a timer. I closed the door so as not to scare my kids too much and told her, through my tears, what I had just read. My voice choked as I held back a sob.

"This is horrifying," I said. "I don't want to think about this stuff."

"It's okay," she said, "I'm here. Go ahead and think about it."

"It's NOT okay."

"Keep crying. We are going to figure this out."

I cried quietly for a few minutes. Then blew my nose. I felt like I was really young.

"I'm tired of being the only one who is hopeful. I'm giving up."

"No, you are not giving up. And you are not the only one who is hopeful. That's bullshit."

"Can't I just sit around and watch sitcoms on TV and eat ice cream like other people do?"

"You are funny."

"Oh God, I HATE this. I'm still scared when people yell at me. I won't do well if there is a war."

"Yes you will. We'll be in it together. Keep crying. I'm right here."

I complained, I protested, and I sobbed.

After a while, I felt my mind starting to settle and clear, as it always does after a good cry with someone who knows not to take your discouragement too seriously.

I stood up and walked around my living room with my portable phone, as reality began to come into focus.

"Jule . . . there have got to be some solutions here."

"I agree."

"I think there must be some way in which we are thinking about this whole thing the wrong way. Technology, profits, petroleum, climate change, now it's people fighting over water . . . everyone is blaming everyone else, and we are still not looking at the whole thing, how it's all interconnected."

She laughed, as the timer went off. "I'm telling you, you are going to figure this out. Just keep reading and talking about it. But next time call me before you get so sunk. Okay?"

"Okay."

"Ready for me?" she asked.

It was my turn to listen as she talked about her life.

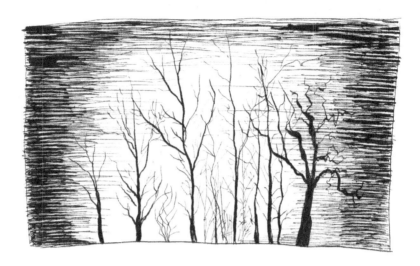

Health Care's Impact on Climate

John Leigh is a brilliant and friendly environmentalist who works in the basement of Dartmouth-Hitchcock Medical Center, in New Hampshire, managing their waste and recycling programs—a huge and important task, suited to someone whose background includes ten years working in the Environmental Protection Agency.

I had visited him the year before to learn about a calculation tool he developed, under a grant from the Maverick Lloyd Foundation, which estimates how much of the Earth's resources a hospital uses (the ecological footprint), as well as how much greenhouse gas a hospital is adding to the environment based on all of its activities (the carbon footprint). While I was there, he had given me a tutorial of how to use the Eco-Health Calculator.[13]

The hospital he works at is a large, modern teaching hospital that has adopted ecologically responsible practices like recycling waste, carpooling, and helping to fund public transport and

---

13 The calculator is available online at https://sites.google.com/site/dhmccalculator/home.

affordable housing nearby for staff. They have been named one of the nation's best hospitals. John had shown me around their massive waste-management department, explaining where all the garbage goes, what is recycled, and what they do with the radio-active waste from CT scans and radiation treatment, and other toxic waste.

He had shown me how Dartmouth-Hitchcock—a 400-bed hospital—uses 83 global hectares of resources every single day. Put another way, each day a patient spends in the hospital uses up six months' worth of his or her annual allotted ecological footprint.[14]

Now I read back through my notes, trying to understand the impact a hospital of that size has on atmospheric carbon.

According to John's calculation tool, if you count the energy usage of Dartmouth-Hitchcock for cooling, heating, and running all the equipment, plus the energy used to manufacture all the supplies, food, drugs, and technology that are used at the hospital, plus the transportation used by staff, patients, and visitors to get to the hospital, plus a few other things like sewage and water, each year of the hospital's activities adds 190,288 metric tons of greenhouse gases (called CO_2 equivalents or "CO_2e") to the atmosphere.

That seemed like a lot to me, but big numbers are often hard to fathom. I wondered what that would look like if I broke it down a little further.

I pulled my own calculator out of the drawer and called my son Alden in to the kitchen. Alden loves numbers. When he was two and I read out loud to him from picture books, he'd ask me to move my hand so he could see the page numbers. When he was three he used to entertain himself by looking at the thermometer and calculating in his head how cold it would be when it went up or down a certain number of degrees from the current temperature.

I handed him the calculator. "Can you help me figure this out?"

"Yessss!" he said enthusiastically.

14 Dartmouth Hitchcock's Eco-health footprint calculator.

"190,288 tons divided by 365 days per year equals what?"

"521.336986301."

"I don't need decimals."

"I like decimals," said Alden.

"I know. So the hospital is emitting about 521 metric tons of carbon dioxide equivalent per *day* . . . Okay . . . This isn't looking good. Now divide that by 400 beds."

"1.30334246575," said Alden.

"1.3? Caring for one patient lying in a bed releases one ton of carbon dioxide rising into the atmosphere *every day*? This can't be right," I said to my son.

The World Health Organization recommends that we aim toward less than two tons of emissions per person per *year*.[15] According to John's numbers, if I spent a week in the hospital I'd be using more than four years' worth of my allotted greenhouse gas emissions.

I called John, who had just come back from a year's sabbatical in which he bicycled around the world with his wife and children. I told him my calculations.

"1.3 metric tons per patient per *day*? This couldn't be right, could it?"

"Unfortunately, it is," he said. "Of course there are also walk-in patients who share the responsibility. Or you could blame it on the staff. If you divide up the total by the 5,360 staff members, you could say each of us who works here is contributing 35.5 metric tons per year, and the patients are just lying there innocently in their beds."

"I think you get some carbon credits, John—you run the recycling program."

"I sure hope so," he said.

15 "Protecting Health from Climate Change," World Health Organization, accessed June 9, 2015, http://www.who.int/world-health-day/previous/2008/toolkit/en/.

⚔

Practice Greenhealth has another energy impact calculation tool (available online)[16] that shows the *cost* of the societal damage associated with a hospital or clinic's energy usage, using the US Environmental Protection Agency's calculations, as well as the medical impact of those pollutants on society. So, for example, a medical facility using 29,488,474 kilowatt-hours per year is responsible for at least 2.5 million dollars' worth of societal damage through annual emissions of carbon dioxide, mercury, sulfur dioxide, and other pollutants from the power plants that create the electricity. That is reflective of their electrical bills alone. Alden and I punched in those numbers to try to put them in terms we could relate to.

It came to a little more than eight cents of societal damage per kilowatt-hour, close to the same price we pay for the electricity itself.

I looked at my son. "Wow," I said. "Modern health care is a high-impact sport."

How Important Is Health Care for Our Health?

Surprisingly, health care isn't really what makes us healthy. In studies of the social determinants of health, the World Health Organization found that professional health care is only responsible for 10 percent of our actual health outcomes. Lifestyle choices, such as food, and whether or not we drink or smoke or play outdoors with our children, are responsible for 51 percent. Our environment is responsible for 19 percent, and our own biology and genetics are responsible for the last 20 percent.[17,18,19]

16 "Energy Impact Calculator," Healthcare Clean Energy Exchange, accessed September 13, 2012, http://www.eichealth.org/docs/eic%20midwestern%20case%20study1.pdf.
17 J. M. McGinnis and W. H. Foege, "Actual Causes of Death in the United States," *JAMA* 270, no. 18 (1993):2207–12, accessed June 9, 2015, http://www.ncbi.nlm.nih.gov/pubmed/8411605.
18 Alvin R. Tarlov, "Public Policy Frameworks for Improving Population Health," *Annals of the New York Academy of Sciences* 896 (1999):281–93.
19 Ali H. Mokdad, et al., "Actual Causes of Death in the United States 2000," *JAMA* 291, no. 10 (2004):1238–45.

Health care is also right up there in causes of death. According to the *Journal of the American Medical Association*, adverse reactions to drugs *properly administered* are estimated to be somewhere between the fourth and sixth leading cause of death in the United States.[20,21] According to one study, standard medicine as a whole—if you take into account medical and pharmaceutical errors, adverse side effects, bedsores, and hospital-acquired infections—is the number one cause of death in the US, higher than heart attacks, car accidents, and cancer.[22]

I began to realize the absurdity of this whole cycle.

Health care is hugely dependent on fossil fuels, and every dollar we spend on things that are made with fossil fuels contributes to climate change. In the United States, we spend substantially more per capita on health care than any other country. It's nearly 18 percent of our GDP. Therefore, as consumers and providers, we are participating in a health-care system that is contributing substantially to the destruction of all the world's delicate ecosystems, which depend upon a uniquely balanced climate for their existence. These are the ecosystems that our bodies evolved in, and are adapted to, for our own health and survival. Is for-profit health care wreaking havoc on our health?

It was like a puzzle.

Does the World Have a Fever?

Let's take a minute and step way, way back.

If I look at the biosphere of the Earth as if I were looking at a patient, I notice that the symptoms—increased temperature, and huge disruptions in the flow and storage of water—are similar to the symptoms of inflammation in the human body.

20 J. Lazarou, et al., "Incidence of Adverse Drug Reactions in Hospitalized Patients: A Meta-analysis of Prospective Studies," *JAMA* 279, no. 15 (1998) 1200–05.
21 Institute of Medicine, "To Err is Human: Building a Safer Health System," 1999.
22 Gary Null, et al., "Death by Medicine," *Life Extension Magazine*, March 2004.

Chronic inflammatory processes are on the rise in our population, and one could say the same is true for our planet. It's a metaphor, but it is worth examining, because in fact we are part of the same system, and parts of a system tend to reflect the whole. What is inflammation? It is the body's normal response to unfamiliar circumstances that threaten to disrupt its functions.

I see the symptoms of climate change as very clear signals that it's time to reevaluate the way we are interacting with the natural systems around us.

We continue to introduce more and more unfamiliar elements into our bodies and into our environment—a nearly constant stream of chemicals (many of them toxic) going into the water, air, vegetation, and soil. Our increasing use of technology disrupts natural processes around us, and changes the relationships between elements (humans, microorganisms, animals, plants, insects, rivers, oceans, etc.). The result is that the systems within us, and around us, are changing as they try to adapt.

As Albert Einstein said, "We can't solve problems using the same thinking we were using when we created them."

The mentality that led us into this unhealthy situation is the reductionist, mechanistic model applied to our inner and outer landscapes. We try to take apart the natural world, figure out who or what is causing a problem, and fix it, or replace it, using technology. It's a strategy that works well with machines. But the Earth is not a machine.

The complexity of natural systems, like our bodies and our planet, is almost unfathomable. All the parts are important, all the parts are interdependent on others, and their actions are changing and shifting constantly in response to what every other part is doing. The carbon cycle that regulates our climate isn't just about fossil fuels and CO_2. The carbon cycle is the unfolding of creation itself: it involves every living thing in the past, present, and future, from the tiniest organisms at the bottom of the ocean to the electrical signals that make our hearts beat.

Any real solutions, therefore, will have to include *all* the parts. On the one hand that may seem like a daunting task, but on the other hand, it means that any lasting solution is likely to help solve the whole thing: flooding, drought, health issues, extinctions, wars over resources, hurricanes, pollution—you name it.

The kind of shift we are looking for is going to involve something hugely creative.

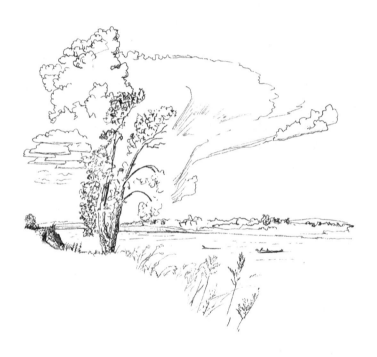

CHAPTER SIX

The Carbon Underground:
The Microbiome of the Soil[1]

"The seeming emptiness of space is an illusion of our limited
sensory capacity, for it is filled with the evanescent tendrils of
yearning that every particle of matter has for all others. There is
no loneliness or isolation in a universe crammed with a matrix
of allurement."

—David Suzuki[2]

I'm talking to my friend Bob about climate change. Bob is a
software engineer and web designer who used to be the repair-
man for the private jet of his Indian guru. He now spends his
weekends building trebuchets, reading history books, and fixing
things, like my vacuum cleaner. When I get overwhelmed, he
invites me over to his house, which is filled with computers, sits
me down in front of his woodstove, and cooks me delicious things
in his microwave.

I point out that over the past century, we have pulled a lot of
carbon out of the ground and sent it into the atmosphere in the
form of CO_2. Now we are trying to solve the climate crisis by figuring out who is to blame. Should we focus on auto emissions, on

1   My friends at The Carbon Underground kindly gave me permission to use their
    trademarked name for this section heading.
2   David T. Suzuki and Amanda McConnell, *The Sacred Balance: A Visual Celebration
    of Our Place in Nature* (Vancouver: Greystone Books, 2002).

power plants, or on feedlots? Should we pressure our politicians or our neighbors?

The more the climate crisis heats up, the more fragmented and bizarre the blame becomes. Recently, the Woods Hole Research Center released a dead-serious article saying that arctic ground squirrels were partially to blame for melting the permafrost layer and worsening global warming. The problem, reported newspapers, is that they dig under the permafrost, and then their urine and feces nourish the microbes that create methane. That same week, other researchers blamed beavers, hypothesizing that their shallow, stagnant beaver ponds allow biological material to build up, which similarly releases methane via the activity of microbes.

Bob points out that even I can play this game: by blaming hospitals, capitalists, and technology. I have to admit that he is right.

We definitely need to stop blaming, and start reducing our fossil fuel emissions. But there is another issue here. Even if we stopped all emissions today, unless we can find a way to actually *remove* the excess CO_2 from the atmosphere, current modeling predicts that temperatures will continue to rise, and will not drop significantly for centuries, or even millennia, because there is a delay in the effect.[3]

It's as if we are filling up a huge bathtub in the sky faster than the drain can work.

So, it's not just about getting people, or squirrels, to stop their behavior. In order to actually *reverse* global warming, we'll have to figure out how to get the excess carbon out of the sky and put it back in the ground. Since the carbon cycle involves all of life, this is a challenge unlike any other. So instead of spending our time trying to find out who is to blame for putting it up there in the first place, we might want to focus on figuring out who is most willing, and who is most capable, to do the work of bringing it back down.

3   Susan Soloman, et al., "Irreversible Climate Change Due to Carbon Dioxide Emissions," Proceedings of the National Academy of Sciences, (2009):106 (6), 1704–09.

Bob puts down a plate of steaming burritos and pulls an oversize container of BJ's guacamole out of the refrigerator.

"I think someone could invent a machine . . . " Bob says, "that takes CO_2 out of the air and breaks it back down into carbon and oxygen."

"That wouldn't work," I say. "You'd need to use some sort of fossil fuel to keep the machine going."

"No you wouldn't," he says. "It would be solar powered."

As it turns out, Bob was right. Shortly after our conversation I learned that "someone" did invent a way to take CO_2 out of the atmosphere, break it back down into carbon stored safely in the soil, and in the process, create oxygen so fresh we can breathe it. The process is powered entirely by sunlight, so it is cheap, and it's not even noisy. Amazing.

But Bob was also wrong, because it wasn't a person who invented the process. Land plants and water-dwelling phytoplankton do this all day long, quietly, freely, without complaint, as if it was their God-given purpose. The process is called photosynthesis, and it has been happening on our planet for more than two billion years.

The carbon cycle on land—a beautiful dance between deep-rooted plants, soil microorganisms, fungi, minerals, sunlight, moisture, and insect and animal life—actually moves carbon out of the atmosphere and very efficiently puts it to work building life on Earth. Photosynthesis is only the first step. Carbon moves first through plant carbohydrates into everything that eats the plants and their sugary exudates, and then moves on out, in multiple directions, through the food chain. Even though we are not plants, we wouldn't be here without photosynthesis.

We often think of carbon simply as something inert and chemical: but carbon is *life*, constituting more than 50 percent of the dry weight of all living organisms. Soil that has been depleted by mismanagement loses the life in it, and therefore has less carbon in it (letting more escape to the atmosphere). Healthy topsoil, on the other hand, is a carbon-rich ecosystem in itself, full of tiny carbon-based life-forms that feed on each other and on the sweet sugary carbon-chain exudates that plant roots give off—up to 40 percent of the sugars that plants make go into the soil to feed microscopic fungi and bacteria. In return, these soil microorganisms provide the carbon-based plants with the soil structures and nutrients they need to grow deep, healthy roots and keep the whole process moving downward, and upward: feeding animals and people as well.

The pathway to deeper and more permanent carbon storage in soils happens through the mycorrhizal fungi that grow on plant roots. These microscopic fungi are beneficial to plants because they act as an extension of a plant's root system—they are shaped like little tubes—and they actively explore the soil to find nutrients and water for the plants. A cubic meter of healthy soil can have up to 25,000 kilometers of these microscopic strands of fungal hyphae—twice the diameter of the Earth. Mycorrhizal fungi also form a glue called glomalin. This sticky stuff binds together particles of sand, silt, and clay, and creates a relatively stable structure—the soil aggregate—in which carbon no longer can oxidize (turn into CO_2), because there is very little oxygen inside. This is how soil carbon accumulates and gets stored at deeper and deeper layers in healthy soils.[4,5,6] The Earth's soils currently store 2,500 billion tons of carbon—more carbon than the atmosphere (780 billion tons) and plants (560 billion tons) combined. But due to mismanagement, soils have lost 50 to 70 percent of their original carbon stores.[7] Carbon isn't the problem: carbon is life. Much of the carbon in the atmosphere came from the soils, where it was doing important work. The problem is that carbon that was in a

4   Walter Jehne, soil microbiologist, private interview, October 2015.

5   Sara Wright, "Glomalin, a Manageable Soil Glue," http://www.ars.usda.gov/sp2UserFiles/Place/12650400/glomalin/brochure.pdf.

6   Douglas L. Godbold, et al., "Mycorrhizal Hyphal Turnover as a Dominant Process for Carbon Input into Soil Organic Matter," *Plant and Soil* 281 (2006):15–24.

7   Rattan, Lal, "Managing Soils and Ecosystems for Mitigating Anthropogenic Carbon Emissions and Advancing Global Food Security," *BioScience* 60.9 (2010): 708–21.

solid form in soils has escaped as a gas, leaving desertified landscapes down below.

So, can we use photosynthesis and soil microbiology to help turn atmospheric carbon back into living and stored carbon on Earth? Yes, we can, and people are already doing it. Certain farmers and ranchers have been experimenting with ways to improve soil carbon formation on the land they are stewarding, so much so that they have been referred to as "carbon cowboys" and "carbon farmers."

However, it's important to understand one thing: ocean ecosystems have already been working overtime to keep our atmospheric carbon lower, by absorbing as much of the excess carbon as they possibly can (a process called "acidification"). So although soil restoration has a huge potential to draw down atmospheric carbon, much of the carbon that the oceans have been holding for us will have to be released back into the atmosphere before we actually see a decrease in parts per million in the atmosphere, or in global temperatures. Since it's going to take a while for the effects to kick in, now would be a good time for us all to learn how to make it actually work, because it's actually not that hard, and there are lots of other benefits (which I'll get to in the next section).

Returning to the bathtub metaphor: in order to stop the overflow of carbon in the great bathtub in the sky (and to lessen the strain on the ocean organisms that are trying desperately to mop up the excess), we need to unplug the drain—and that will involve restoring ecosystems so that plants, trees, and soil organisms can use the power of photosynthesis to take atmospheric CO_2 and put that carbon back into creative use: rebuilding the underground structures that we all depend on for health and resilience, rather than storing it in a vault somewhere as if it was radioactive waste.

I called Bob up and told him what I had learned.

"Huh!" he said, sounding vaguely interested. "But I still want to invent a machine that will do the same thing. That would be *really* cool."

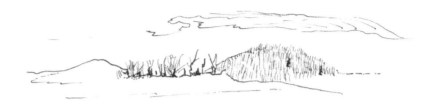

Healthy Soil Can Store and Filter Water

Even though it may be a while before we get to witness the impact of soil restoration on atmospheric carbon levels, it's not as if there aren't immediate benefits to restoring soil ecology.

Plants and soil microorganisms, if allowed to do their work, create underground structures that hold soil particles together in a huge porous "carbon sponge" of stable aggregates. As rainwater filters slowly through this carbon sponge and into wells and rivers, it is naturally filtered, becoming clear and clean for human and animal consumption. The plants like it too.

When this carbon sponge is allowed to form at deeper and deeper layers, it doesn't just hold more carbon in the earth; it also can hold much more water in the earth, in the pore spaces between soil aggregates, and this dramatically lessens the tendency toward both flooding and drought—important in our new climate. When water does flood an area that has healthy topsoil, soil doesn't erode as easily, and river banks are less likely to crumble and wash away.

Soil aggregates are those little clumps that you see in healthy soil, especially around the roots of healthy plants. That's where mycorrhizal fungi and other microorganisms tend to congregate because that's where plants are giving off free sugars in exchange for services.

Well-aggregated soil is like bread—full of tiny pockets of air space—so rain sinks in more quickly, and evaporates more slowly. Unaggregated soil is like flour: water just runs off, and erodes the particles. To get an idea of what happens when rain hits unaggregated soil, try pouring a cup of water onto a pile of flour. Then, to see what happens when rain hits aggregated soil, try pouring a cup of water onto some slices of bread. You'll see why, in landscapes where soil has been allowed to develop aggregates, flooding and drought are less likely to happen.

The Intelligence of Soils

As I mentioned earlier when writing about Ted's farm, mycorrhizal fungi have another crucial role to play. Walter Jehne, a soil microbiologist from Australia who researched the structure and functions of healthy soil, has helped me understand the innate intelligence that resides in healthy soils, and how that intelligence impacts our health:

The higher fungi are actual proto-animals in their genetic heritage, and they have similar nutritional needs. According to Jehne, when mycorrhizal fungi search out nutrients they act as intelligent filters. As they move through the soil, they are actively seeking out, selecting, and absorbing essential nutrients at the right *concentrations*, in the right *forms*, in the right *ratios*, and in the right *balances*. At the same time, they are excluding overdoses of toxic nutrients. This ability to discriminate between necessary and harmful substances is actually what makes life possible: it is the defining function of the membrane of every cell, including the first single-celled organism. Mycorrhizal fungi are like a huge membrane in the soil: an intelligent interface between the chemical, inert, toxic, mineral soil and the living healthy cytoplasm of life. This has benefits for the fungi themselves, obviously, but because they bring these nutrients to plants, it also has benefits for the rest of the ecosystem around them. One cubic meter of healthy soil can have 25,000 kilometers of fungal hyphae. That's twice the diameter of the Earth, and that's a lot of work being done for the organisms that live there.

Plants are essentially symbiotic organisms. Most plants have evolved to depend on fungi to help find and select nutrients for them,[8] and protect them from toxins, not unlike the way we, as animals, depend on our gut and skin microorganisms to aid and protect us. As animals who eat plants, however, we also depend on mycorrhizal fungi to filter our own nutrients, because as we eat those plants, we take in whatever nutrients the plant took in.

The nutritional integrity of foods grown in a setting where nutrients can be taken up from the soil in this discriminating way is fundamentally different from the nutritional integrity of food that has been produced without this intelligent filter.

In industrial soils, where mycorrhizal fungi have been killed off by tillage, fungicides, and other chemicals, there is no intelligent cytoplasmic filter to discriminate what balance of nutrients is appropriate for sustaining life. Instead, the plants are left to their own devices in a man-made chemical soup awash in fertilizers, herbicides, pesticides, fungicides, and non-living mineral particles. Those mineral particles are often negatively charged, so the nutrients available are often the anions, the nitrates, phosphates, chlorine—soluble nutrients—which include a lot of toxic substances. Plants growing in this man-made soup suck up huge amounts of nitrogen, phosphorus, and potassium that have been added through chemical fertilizers, along with indiscriminate amounts of arsenic, lead, nitrates, sulfates, chlorine, and whatever else is in the soils.

Meanwhile, plants in industrial fields also have no help in finding or accessing other, less available but essential nutrients like selenium, zinc, and magnesium. Yet those are precisely the nutrients that plants, animals, and people use to create the enzymes necessary to stay healthy, regulate our biochemistry, and fight off disease.

Plants in industrial systems are becoming less resilient: increasingly dependent on highly profitable chemical applications to ward off diseases and pests. People are also becoming less resilient, and

8   With a few exceptions: most notably the brassica family of broccoli, kale, and cabbages.

Carbon Cycling in the Ocean

At least 25 percent of the CO_2 released by burning fossil fuels ends up in the oceans, where it is cycled in various ways. Water-dwelling plants, called phytoplankton (including cyanobacteria, or "blue-green algae"), perform photosynthesis and break down CO_2 into oxygen and carbon, just like the plants on land do. In fact, it was through this process that phytoplankton formed the oxygen that made life on Earth possible in the first place, and they continue to produce approximately half of all the oxygen on our planet. When they die, shelled phytoplankton and zooplankton shuttle some of that carbon down to deep storage at the bottom of the ocean as they sink, which may be how the deep-sea stores of petroleum were formed.

Cyanobacteria are found in vast quantities in oceans, but also in freshwater, soils, and hot springs. Some are found as symbiotic partners of lichens and fungi, and even in the fur of sloths. It appears that 1.5 billion years ago they partnered with other organisms in symbiotic relationships and became light-absorbing chloroplasts, which eventually allowed terrestrial plants to have the capacity to perform photosynthesis, as well.

Much of the CO_2 that ends up in the ocean is not processed by phytoplankton; instead it dissolves and forms carbonic acid, changing the pH of the oceans. The recent increase in acidity in the oceans (acidification) due to increased CO_2 emissions is causing problems for marine life-forms that cannot adapt fast enough to the change in pH. The carbonic acid dissolves calcium-based shells and corals, the same way vinegar can dissolve the minerals that collect in your coffee pot.

If we can successfully draw down CO_2 from the atmosphere, the oceans will release some of their CO_2 (like a soda bottle with the top off). This will lessen the stresses on oceans, but also lengthen the time we have to wait to see the drop in parts per million in the atmosphere that we are trying to achieve. Luckily there are many ways in which soil restoration can help offset the effects of climate change on land while the oceans restore their own balance.

more dependent on pharmaceutical drugs. Our food now has less than one-third of the nutrient density it had pre–World War II, and often none of the rarer essential nutrients. Jehne sums it up nicely: "We are starving ourselves with our industrial food system."[9]

Soil microorganisms, though they are invisible to us, play a huge role in our lives. They influence not only the carbon cycle and the water cycle, but they also have a profound influence on the cycling of nutrients as well. We are dependent on healthy, intelligent, living soils for our atmosphere, our safety, and our own health.

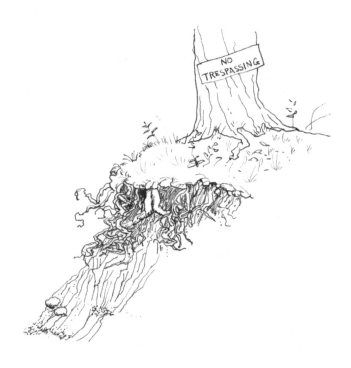

9   This whole section on the intelligence of soils reflects several long conversations with Walter Jehne when he came to visit me after the "Restoring Water Systems to Reverse Global Warming" conference at Tufts University in October 2015.

The Soil Carbon Challenge

"The biosphere is the sum of all the living and the dead. It doesn't just sit there looking pretty, wild, or vulnerable. It does work, a lot of it . . . The issue [with rising atmospheric carbon levels] is not just technology, though it plays a large role. The issue is that, over vast areas of the world, the biosphere is not doing enough work. With livestock confined, and crop monocultures dependent on fossil energy to maintain them, too many of the animals are in prison, too many of the plants are on welfare, and too many of the microbes are dead."

—**Peter Donovan**, *Measuring Soil Carbon Change*[10]

In the summer of 2014, the Northeast Organic Farming Association hosted a special series of workshops on soil carbon at their annual summer conference. I was so excited I could hardly contain myself. I had been reading and learning everything I could about it, but now I had three days to completely immerse myself.

I learned to differentiate bacteria, fungi, and nematodes under a microscope. I learned about forest gardens, cover cropping, and biochar. I square danced with farmers, and stayed up late laughing with a new group of friends. On the very last day there was one workshop left in the soil-carbon track that didn't sound that interesting. It was called "Monitoring Soil Carbon Data," and I thought maybe I'd skip it.

But I had a vague recollection that the teacher, Peter Donovan, might be the man I had read about who had sold his belongings except for his piano, and was traveling the country in a school bus, measuring soil carbon.[11]

---

10 Peter Donovan, "Measuring Soil Carbon Change: A Flexible, Practical, Local Method," http://www.soilcarboncoalition.org/files/MeasuringSoilCarbonChange.pdf.
11 Judith Schwartz profiled Peter Donovan in the first chapter of her book *Cows Save the Planet: and Other Improbable Ways of Restoring Soil to Heal the Earth* (White River Junction, VT: Chelsea Green, 2013). This is the wonderfully written book that first taught me about soil carbon. When I finished the book, I decided on the spot to devote the second half of my life to soil restoration.

I decided to check it out.

I walked into a room where a group of people was pushing chairs around, helter-skelter. A rugged-looking older man who looked way too conservative to live in a school bus was trying to direct them. "Please put your chairs in a circle," he was saying. But they weren't. "No," he said, slowly, "not in *two* rows, I want *one* circle where we can all see each other." Someone protested that there wasn't enough space.

He paused, and then spoke even more slowly. "We spend enough of our days in hierarchical power structures. I don't want that in this room."

Everyone, including me, stopped talking, made a circle, and sat down as if a huge game of musical chairs was just ending.

"Now," said Peter, "Tell me why you are here and what you hope to learn."

As we went around the room, everyone had things they wanted to know about how to get more carbon in the ground through their apple orchards, dairy operations, forests, and gardens. I wanted to know if I should cut down my pine trees and get some goats.

"I'm sorry. I can't answer any of those questions. We just don't know enough yet."

He explained that the carbon cycle is a huge topic and we have almost no data, other than synthetic data (in which someone takes a small piece of information and tries to extrapolate how it might pan out on a broad scale). He explained that people are afraid to try things for themselves. They just want the answers, from experts, in the form of modeling, predictions, policies, and practices. Yet without real data, we can't compare real outcomes and find the people whose land management is creating the best results in a particular region.

"Data works on our imaginations," he said. "It can change our ideas and open our minds to what is possible. That's why we started the Soil Carbon Challenge. Each of you is farming on land that is unique. So, be creative, try things, monitor the results, and then tell me what you discover. Today, instead of telling you what to do, I'm going to talk to you about the seven generations of sunlight, and why the carbon cycle is the most powerful and creative planetary force. Maybe that will give you some ideas.

"The carbon cycle," he began, "is not really about carbon. It is about sunlight energy stored in chemical bonds. We think of the carbon cycle as a movement of material, but it is also a flow of energy over time, which means it is about power, and work, which are processes. We don't understand it easily because we don't deal with processes well. As a society, we are focused more on things. The whole system we live in is actually a flow—not a collection of things. The only way we can make good decisions is by closely observing the effects we are having on this constantly flowing system. It's like watching the way the water flow changes when we place rocks in a running stream."

I started writing notes, fast. His view of the Earth struck me as remarkably similar to the way I was trained, as an acupuncturist, to view the body—as a series of flows of various functions. Physics, chemistry, and biology were spinning in my brain.

"Let's look at it in terms of work." He drew a graph with three bars.

"This . . . "—he drew a smokestack on top of the shortest bar—"is the amount of work that all the fossil fuels we burn are performing.

"This . . . "—he drew a volcano on top of the next-highest bar—"is the amount of work that geologic forces do—shifting continents, earthquakes, volcanoes. It can be slow, or it can be dramatic, but we don't have much control over it.

"And *this* . . . "—he drew an elephant on top of the tallest bar, which was much higher than both the others—"is the amount of work that the biosphere does, through photosynthesis, the water cycle, and other forms of biological work. It's hard for us to imagine the potential of soil and plants to move CO_2 out of the atmosphere, because our technology appears so powerful, and it seems to be creating so much more change, so much faster. *But the biosphere moves nine times the carbon and does nine times the work of all fossil-fuel burning.*"

His hour-long talk described the flow of sunlight's energy and influence on the world, all the way from photosynthesis to human consciousness, and then he reminded us of our current ability— through the decisions we make—to affect the cycle of carbon and water, and all the life that flows from them, for better or for worse.

He ended by inviting us to join the monitoring process he was doing—testing soil, and tracking changes in the accumulation of soil carbon over time—on land managed by farmers and ranchers trying innovative things to figure out what worked best in their regions. He didn't mention a school bus. He didn't actually say much of anything about himself.

As we went around the circle again, answering his question— what did you learn, and what do you want to do about it?—the other participants seemed disappointed that he hadn't answered their questions. Some people protested that there wasn't time to monitor changes: we had to do something about the climate, *now.*

Peter seemed unperturbed by their urgency.

I followed him out of the class and down the stairs. "Where do you come to this work from—are you a soil biologist?"

"No," he said.

"Oh . . . what *did* you study. I mean, what's your academic background?"

"Classical music, and languages."

I digested that for a few minutes.

"You were in Judy Schwartz's book about soil restoration, weren't you? You are the guy with the school bus?"

"Yes."

I remembered reading Judy's description of the bus, with a piano in it.

I also remembered saying to myself, somewhere in the middle of reading Judy's book, when I first began to understand the huge creative potential of soil restoration, *"This is what I'm going to devote the second half of my life to."* A simultaneous realization and vow.

As Peter and I walked outside, his tendency toward silence gave me a chance to reflect. I had been an acupuncturist for more than twenty years, but my sense of what it meant to be a health-care provider had been shifting. First it was a different economic outlook: I had moved into my clinic and changed my practice to a more economically viable one, for me and my patients. Then, through my own kitchen, nutrient-dense food had become more central to my practice, and I started to think about food production as part of health care. In 2011, the flooding from Irene turned my Ompompanoosuc River into a torrent, and swept me into the real-ization that climate change was all about water, with huge impli-cations for public health. Now, something even larger was turning inside me. The more I learned about the carbon and water cycles, the more the systems of the body and those of the Earth were start-ing to merge in my mind.

I felt like a boat, facing a steady, insistent wind that was pushing me in a whole new direction. Maybe my practice was really too limited, given what I was trying to accomplish. Treating human health, without addressing the health of the land, was starting to feel like yet another version of the sterile, disconnected, "specialist" mentality. But was I really going to devote the second half of my life to soil and water? There was so much to learn. Was I going to start again at zero, as a beginner? What about my patients? What about the practice I had built up?

Peter's way of viewing our current challenges and opportunities sat well with my own. His project seemed like something I could get involved in, without going back for another degree. But I was a single parent, with a busy health-care practice, teaching classes in the evenings, and with an overdue, unfinished book project. I knew

if I took on another project, something would have to give, and I
didn't know what it would be.

I loved my life . . .

My sweet, little, local life.

I took a deep breath.

"I'd like you to train me to do soil monitoring."

Peter stopped, and finally looked straight into my eyes. "I'll be on
the East Coast for the next two weeks," he said. "You tell me a time."

⚔

Two months later, Peter and I were in Saskatchewan, Canada,
hanging out with ranchers, helping to move cattle, and remon-
itoring some of the earliest test plots Peter had put in, at five
holistically managed ranches. I was photographing and filming
the process so that the organization he founded, the Soil Carbon
Coalition, could train more people to monitor changes in the
soil, and I was beginning to piece together some ideas to get
schools involved. The goal was to start connecting the dots while
creating an online "Atlas of Biological Work"—a multilayered
mapping system, tracking changes over time in photosynthesis,
flows of water, productivity per inch of rainfall, accumulation of
soil carbon, and other changes in landscape functions and flows.
The atlas would serve as an open database and social network for
people involved in land-restoration projects and monitoring. As
we filled in the map with actual data, we would be able to identify those places on Earth where the biosphere is doing the best
work, and by extension, identify and learn from the people who
are successfully restoring the ecological functions of the land they
are stewarding.

The revolution in land-management policies, says Peter, should
be led by these people—the outliers—the most creative and successful land managers. But we can't find them without the data.

Carbon Cowboys

> "Every blade of grass has its angel that bends
> over it and whispers, 'Grow, grow.'"
> —the Talmud

As we traveled together for the week, I learned that Peter had lived outdoors on sheep ranches in semi-wild Oregon, working in partnership with dogs and mules rather than people. This helped explain his rather terse conversation style, and his relative ease with not having a home. It also explained his deep, almost religious love for the land, and his view of all life as an evolutionary flow of sunlight.

While working on ranches, he took a workshop on holistic decision making with Allan Savory, one of the pioneers of soil restoration, and it changed the course of his life.

In the 1960s, Savory had been working on the interrelated problems of increasing poverty, desertification, and disappearing wildlife in Rhodesia, Africa. After many failed efforts (mostly involving excluding animals from the landscape to allow grass to regrow—which, instead, led to even faster desertification), Savory decided to research healthy grassland ecosystems and see if he could reproduce what was happening there. Grasslands, it turned out, had evolved together with grazing animals, and predators. Savory decided to try using carefully managed herds of cattle to mimic the natural movement of wild grazing animals.

Following the patterns of wild herds, he would move the cattle frequently to new parcels of land, keeping them closely bunched together as if there were predators all around, and wouldn't bring them back to the same spot for many months.

As he moved them through the cracked, desertified landscape, Savory found that the animals' hooves broke through the crusts, pushing seeds into the ground and creating pockets where rain could collect. They trampled old dead plants, flattening them to the ground and creating soil cover that helped keep the soil cooler, kept moisture from evaporating, and created habitat for beneficial soil microorganisms to grow. As the animals moved through an area, their manure and nitrogen-rich urine also added microorganisms and nutrients to the soil, exactly what was needed to promote new growth.

It worked. Within just one season, grasses began to reappear—even in the dry, cracked soils of Africa—slowly at first, but within two years, quite lushly. As time went on, on parcels managed in this way, dried-out riverbeds started flowing again, new plants sprang up everywhere, and insects, birds, and other animals returned.

More than fifteen villages in the Hwange region around the Africa Centre for Holistic Management in Zimbabwe have shifted to large-scale systems of communal grazing, using a group planning and decision-making process for land management. This has had an enormously beneficial outcome for the animals, plants, and people sharing close to 200,000 acres of restored land. In a landscape often associated with starvation, the villagers have created rich topsoil for growing vegetables and fruits, produced healthy animals that yield more meat and dairy products, and dramatically increased the amount of grass and water available for the grazing animals who are key to the whole process. The Dimbangombe River is a full mile longer during the dry season. At the same time, they are lessening the effects of climate change, by restoring small water cycles, and by moving more carbon into the soil.

This process of land restoration creates more life, food, and health, exponentially—just the opposite of the exponential loss that happens in an extractive economy.

Africa isn't the only place with deteriorating grasslands and a resulting loss of carbon-rich topsoil.

In 1935, Congress passed the Soil Conservation Act, partly in response to the Dust Bowl, which affected 100 million acres of US land and sent clouds of black dust all the way to the East Coast. The Dust Bowl was the result of two factors: First, the genocide of huge herds of buffalo (with which the perennial grasses, ecology, and indigenous cultures of the Midwestern plains had evolved). The second factor was that settlers were trying to practice a European style of farming—plowing up the grasslands and planting annual crops—in a seasonally dry landscape that needed constant deep perennial roots in the ground to maintain soil structure and moisture. The US was not alone in this mistake. Over the past 150 years we have lost half of the world's topsoil,[12, 13] due to the use of agricultural techniques that are inappropriate for the landscapes they are used in.

Along with that, we have lost the microorganisms responsible for the structure and function of the soil, which includes the filtration, storage, and distribution of water throughout the landscape. As soil ecology fails, carbon from these life-forms escapes from the land and enters the atmosphere as CO_2, contributing as much as one-third of our global emissions, and dramatically changing the capacity of soils to hold water or produce food.

FDR wrote, "A nation that destroys its soils, destroys itself." In that same letter, he created soil conservation districts across the country, and—for a while—people in government and civil agencies understood, taught, and wrote about soil conservation and grassland ecology. But when the chemical revolution happened in agriculture, in the 1940s and '50s, the natural ecology of soils drifted out of the conversation. From then on, the focus has been on products, not processes. Soil testing, for example, has become a way of determining what chemical you need to buy, and how much of it to add.

This parallels what happened in medicine: profits and products influenced our evaluation, management, and care of our inner and outer landscape. Now we need to return to understanding and restoring *processes*. Topsoil is a delicate mucosal membrane, filled with intelligent organisms, just like our guts are.

12 "Global Desertification Vulnerability Map," USDA National Resources Conservation Service, accessed June 9, 2015, http://www.nrcs.usda.gov/wps/portal/nrcs/detail/national/nedc/training/soil/?cid=nrcs142p2_054003.
13 "Soil Erosion and Degradation," World Wildlife Fund, accessed June 9, 2015, https://www.worldwildlife.org/threats/soil-erosion-and-degradation.

The Body of the Earth

If we think of the Earth as a body, the topsoil is the skin, lungs, and digestive system. In humans, as I discussed earlier, the microbiomes of the skin, respiratory system, and large intestine work together as the *wei qi* or "protective system" of the body. I like to think of topsoil as the mucosal membrane and *wei qi* of the land: a microorganism-filled area, rich in mucosal exudates, providing a layer of protection for life's many processes, including growth and development, exchange of oxygen and other gasses, breakdown and assimilation of nutrients, and creation of new life.

Like our gut bacteria, soil microorganisms also contribute to the "mood" of the land: the types of plants, animals, and insects that appear in a particular niche within a landscape are very much determined by who is living underground. And naturally, it goes both ways: the plants, animals, and insects within a landscape also determine the "mood" and ecology of the soil.[*] The more biodiversity of plants, animals, and insects there is above ground, the more healthy and biologically diverse soil ecology is below ground.[†]

[*]   Elaine Ingham, Keynote Lecture at the Northeast Organic Farming Association Summer Conference, Amherst, Massachusetts, August 8–10, 2014.
[†]   David U. Hooper, et al., "Interactions between Aboveground and Belowground Biodiversity in Terrestrial Ecosystems: Patterns, Mechanisms, and Feedbacks," *BioScience* 50, no. 12 (2000):1049–61.

Peter Donovan once asked a man who had worked at the Soil Conservation Service for years, "What happened? Why did the Conservation Service let go of its mission?"

The man's reply was poetic: "We quit dancing with the girl we brought."

☀

Intact grasslands and forests do a phenomenal job of storing and cycling carbon. But our current agricultural practices—of deforestation, frequent tillage, and heavy application of chemicals—do just the opposite. As trees are cut and grasslands are turned into croplands, soil processes are disrupted over and over again. In the bare, frequently tilled soil of large industrial farms, microorganisms are exposed to high temperatures, die off, and release large amounts of CO_2, without any plants nearby to reabsorb it. Soil, in these conditions, loses its moisture-holding structures and natural carbon-storing properties.

When we introduce heavy agricultural machinery into natural systems like prairies, the underground structures are broken apart. The carbon-based life-forms die off, depleting short-term carbon stores in the soil, and deeper stores of soil carbon cannot continue to form without the deep-rooted perennial grasses and mycorrhizal fungi to shuttle it into the ground.

Although tilling appears to temporarily fluff up the uppermost layer of soil, compaction from heavy machinery actually makes soil aggregates collapse—so the porous structure of the soil is lost, and water and air cannot flow through it. Without air or water, underground life suffers. Crops become more susceptible to pests and disease. The soil dries out, the sticky slimes and glues and fungal hyphae that hold soil in place disappear, and farmers are left with a powdery, dead substance instead of actual living soil. Rains and irrigation wash the dirt downstream, and when a high wind comes through, the dirt just blows away.[14,15]

The topsoil also suffers at large ranches where grazing animals are allowed to roam freely with no predators to keep them moving and bunching together, or in places like national parks that are

14   Don Reicosky, "Tillage and Planting: Impact on Carbon and Soil Quality," http://www.fairfieldswcd.org/Attachments/Soil%20Quality.pdf.
15   Elaine Ingham, Keynote Lecture at the Northeast Organic Farming Association Summer Conference, Amherst, Massachusetts, August 8–10, 2014.

fenced off and "protected" from grazing altogether. The less-tasty, ungrazed, dead plants from previous years shade out the new growth, the tall grasses dry out and can easily catch fire, and the soil gradually forms a crust that rain can't penetrate, leading to flash floods, dramatically higher surface temperatures,[16] erosion, and ultimately, dry, canyon-like riverbeds.[17]

Traditional geologists say soil is a "nonrenewable resource" because it takes hundreds, or even thousands, of years for the Earth to create one centimeter of soil, through the weathering of rocks. That *would* be a frightening fact, given that we are losing 50,000 square kilometers of soil each year—an area the size of Costa Rica.[18] But we now know that we don't have to wait for centuries to create fertile soil. With proper management, we can restore fertility to desertified land and create new topsoil in a matter of just a few years.

Savory's work using grazing animals to restore healthy ecosystems in Africa has inspired land managers around the world to use the same sort of approach—mimicking healthy systems, tracking the progress, and altering it as needed—to keep restoring land to its healthiest, most fertile state. The more biological diversity, the better. That's what the farmers Peter and I visited in Saskatchewan were doing, although the landscape around them was quite different from the cracked earth of Africa.

As we drove down nearly empty roads in Saskatchewan, we saw mile after mile of wheat fields that were gray with mud. It was a familiar sight to me, in a new place. Saskatchewan and neighboring North Dakota had experienced severe flooding earlier that

---

16 Dan Dagget, November 5, 2014, "Global Warming, See for Yourself," dandagget. com, http://www.dandagget.com/global-warming-see-for-yourself.

17 Levente Czegledi and Andrea Radacsi, "Overutilization of Pastures by Livestock," University of Debrecen Centre for Agricultural Studies, http://www.agr.unideb. hu/kiadvany/gyep/2005-03/06Czegledi.pdf.

18 "Soils: The Principal Ally for Feeding the World," The World Bank, accessed June 9, 2015, http://www.worldbank.org/en/news/feature/2015/03/09/suelos-princi pales-aliados-alimentar-planeta.

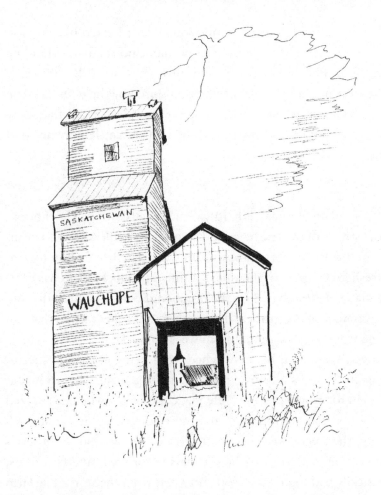

summer. There was little harvesting going on; the fields were quiet, except for the creak of pumping oil rigs that dotted the landscape. Everyone we met explained that seeds on these large industrial farms simply wouldn't germinate that year—they were rotting in the soggy ground. Each farmer tried digging ditches to drain his fields, which led to conflicts with neighboring farmers who didn't want the excess water, either. These were prairie soils that should have had superbly deep topsoil and some of the best drainage in the world. But after a hundred years of heavy tillage and chemical agriculture, the soils were compacted and there was hardly any drainage at all.

Then we'd reach a quarter-mile square that looked like an oasis of green grasses and wildflowers—no mud; no stagnant, standing water; no stubble of old dead plant stalks. These were the farms that were practicing holistic management, inspired by the work of Allan Savory. These were the "soil carbon cowboys" who said they were growing soil, grass, and microbes, and that the cattle were just part of the process.

⤢

Our host, Blain Hjertaas, is hardly your typical cowboy. He unhooks a short strand of electric fence and stands there, allowing 120 beautiful multicolored cows and calves to walk eagerly past him toward the fresh green grass of their next planned paddock. Blain has carefully mapped it out based on the number of cows, the maturity and sugar content of the grasses, the weather, and other factors that can change from day to day, and from week to week.

Fifteen years ago, Blain switched from being a grain farmer to raising cattle and sheep using holistic management, also known as "planned rotational grazing." He made the switch when he realized that the soil was getting more and more compacted, it didn't smell healthy, the weeds were becoming harder to kill, and profit levels were declining. With what he was paying for seeds and chemicals, he basically had to buy the crop every year from the store. The farm itself had been in his family for generations, since they had immigrated to Saskatchewan from Norway.

He reattaches the strand of wire as the last cow passes him. "Well, that's about it for the next couple of days. Pretty tough job, eh?"

I duck under the wire and walk behind the cows, snapping pictures. I don't want it to be over. Somehow I had imagined riders on horses with lassos and a lot of commotion and dust. But this is the calmest ranch scene you could imagine. The birds are singing in the trees next to us. The pond doesn't have a ripple.

Blain can see that I was hoping for something more. "Had enough, or do you want some more?"

"Can we stay a little longer, and just hang out?" I ask. "I need a cow fix."

"Go ahead, have fun. I've got nothing else to do today," he says.

I follow the cows up to the small pond ringed with trees, which looks almost indigo blue as it reflects the late October sky, and then down to the banks of a small river just over a bluff. Around me are thigh-high grasses and forbs, in a dazzling mix of greens, from rich to silvery light, as well as a few wildflowers as if thrown in for color.

The cows—their thick fur polka-dotted and geographically mapped in a circus parade of silvers, blacks, reddish browns, and whites—aren't moving fast; they are too busy eating. The sound around me is not the sound of galloping hooves. There is no bellowing or mooing. Instead, it is the most amazingly loud and satisfying munching noise. There is a rhythm to it: three pulls of ripping grass, echoing slightly through the well-aggregated soils underfoot, then a round of angular chewing and breathing in the cool misty air, with an occasional satisfied thump of a hoof. I sit down, and watch, and listen, and feel my whole nervous system relaxing into some ancient place of comfort.

Later that evening, after Peter finishes giving a talk, I'm standing around with several ranchers at the local meeting hall.

"You know that sound . . ." says an older guy, "of a bunch of cows on fresh grass?"

"Oh my God, it's the best!" I say. "I helped Blain move some cows this morning and afterward I just sat there next to their noses for about an hour, in total bliss."

Everyone laughs, and nods.

"I could fall asleep to it," says another, younger guy, wearing a white cowboy hat and glasses. "There is nothing as relaxing as that sound."

"Ahhhh . . ." says another, tall and lean, throwing his head back.

"Gomph gomph gomph." We all try to imitate it, but it's impossible. Our mouths don't have the sonorous depth, our nostrils aren't big enough, and our teeth aren't flat enough.

"I think we should record it and make some of those relaxation tapes," jokes the guy with the hat.

"And sell them to stressed-out people in the States!"

"Yes! Would they *buy* them?" They all turn to me, giggling.

"Like hotcakes!" I say, thinking of all my patients.

They burst out laughing.

"What would we call it?"

"'Pastoral Pleasures.'"

We all snort.

I catch Peter's eye, across the room. He's having a quiet, serious conversation with another rancher, but he smiles at me with his eyes, clearly pleased to see that I am enjoying myself.

I can't believe how much fun I'm having. I am outside most of the day, spending my evenings laughing with these cowboys, then having deep conversations about the biology, chemistry, and physics of the transition from industrial to restorative farming with Peter, and feeling like I'm participating in restoring health—of people, and all other species—on a much larger level.

Even though I love my work at my clinic, I think back to all the years I've been working only indoors, feeling responsible for all the decisions and care, instead of working in concert with the earth, rain, sun, and animals. I love my patients, but it's like I've been trapped and starved, and so have they.

☒

On each of the five different ranches we visited, Peter, Blain, and I dug down with our trowels and probes into the body of the earth. The oil rigs in the distance moved up and down, keeping time, like metronomes, as we dug. Under the lush grass, we found beautiful well-aggregated soils, with lots of pore space for water and oxygen. We labeled the samples to be sent off to the lab. We did infiltration tests and timed the water moving down into the soil. We measured bare soil, counted the various grass species that were

The Many Accomplishments of Biological Work

Plants, microorganisms, insects, and animals are constantly working to regenerate vibrant, productive landscapes. Their "biological work" is already accomplishing many of the tasks we haven't figured out how to do for ourselves:

- Providing clean drinking water and addressing global water shortages
- Rebuilding fertile, productive soils
- Attracting pollinators and soil-building insects like earthworms and dung beetles
- Eliminating the need for chemical interventions in agriculture
- Increasing local food security
- Providing a wide variety of nutrient-dense foods with more vitamins and minerals, less pesticide residue, and less antibiotic residue
- Decreasing agricultural runoff into rivers, lakes, and oceans
- Preventing conflicts over resources
- Providing the conditions that support biologically diverse plant, animal, microbial, and fungal life
- Absorbing CO_2 from the atmosphere, and putting it to work on the land
- Reducing the impact of climate change by:
  - Creating stable soils that won't get washed away in floods
  - Keeping moisture in soils and vegetation to prevent drought and wildfires
  - Keeping water cycling in local landscapes rather than contributing to ocean rise
  - Cooling the surrounding landscape and stabilizing weather patterns through transpiration

growing within a predetermined hoop, and noted the native ones reappearing.

We lay facedown on the earth with the ranchers and looked at the tiny bugs on the grass with a magnifying loupe, just for fun. We admired the beautiful animals, who needed no grain to fatten them up, no antibiotics to keep them healthy. We sat around after testing and drank tea, or whiskey, with the ranchers. But we didn't know about the carbon. Peter had waited a full three years to come back to these spots, and in the meantime he had travelled 30,000 miles, doing baseline plots on 270 other sites around North America.

Peter and I are talking on Skype. He's back in Oregon, near where he used to herd sheep. He looks up at me, slightly embarrassed. "I know, I know. I am weeping at an Excel spreadsheet. But this is . . . huge. I've only had baselines so far. This is what I've been waiting for. It was starting to feel like . . ." He can't finish the sentence.

"I know," I say. "I understand. It's been a long haul."

I'm savoring this moment: letting this man, who is becoming very dear to me, weep tears of relief on my virtual shoulder . . . and I'm also getting curious. He's waited patiently for three years, but I'm a different breed. Ever since he texted me that the soil test results were in, I've been waiting to know what he's found out. "So . . ." I try to keep my voice calm, "what are the numbers?"

Peter looks up from the papers he has laid out on the counter. "All five," he says to me, wiping the tears from his eyes. "All five farms in Saskatchewan showed a substantial increase in soil carbon on at least two of the layers we sampled. I thought the results would be good, but nothing like this. Blain's average went from 4.09 to 4.57 percent, Neil Dennis from 3 to 3.81. Corcorans from 3.08 to 3.99 . . ."

As he reads down the list, my eyes fill with tears, as well. For I know that these numbers represent not just carbon, but also water—many thousands of gallons of additional water that each acre of land will hold.[19] No wonder their fields and homes were fine during the recent flooding when everyone around them was slogging through mud.

A few weeks later, Blain emails me with some figures he has calculated from the soil data we collected. At Blain's farm each hectare (about the size of a city block) is gaining an average of 6.18 metric tons of carbon each year, while removing almost 23 tons of CO_2[20] from the atmosphere.

That means the entire 320-hectare farm (about 1.2 square miles) is turning the equivalent of 382 Canadian citizens' annual CO_2 emissions each year into fertile soil for growing deep-rooted prairie grass, beautiful wildflowers, fruits and vegetables, and beneficial microorganisms, as well as hundreds of healthy animals: cattle, sheep, pigs, chickens, and turkeys. The restored soil also provides Blain's family with flood protection, clean filtered water, and twenty times more profit than growing wheat.

But Blain's numbers weren't even the best of the five farms we sampled. Not far away, his friends the Corcorans gained a whopping 13.19 tons of carbon per hectare each year—more than twice as much as Blain's land—and five to ten times more than what one would expect based on the little data that has been available from past soil-carbon studies of holistically managed grasslands.[21]

These are just the first numbers. Over the next several years, as the test results of the Soil Carbon Coalition's "Soil Carbon Challenge" come in, we'll be able to compare data from people working to restore function and fertility to land in the rocky hillsides of New England, the drought-ridden fields of California, the flat compacted soils of the Midwest, the hot dry deserts of

19 The absolute increase in percentage of carbon over a three-year period in the plots we sampled ranged from .40 to .91 percent. For every 1 percent increase in soil carbon, it's estimated that the land will hold an additional 15,400 gallons of water per acre. H. D. Scott, L. S. Wood, and W. M. Miley, 1986, "Long-Term Effects of Tillage on the Retention and Transport Of Soil Water," Arkansas Water Resources Research Center Pub. No. 125, 39.
20 A metric ton is about 2,205 pounds.
21 Rattan Lal, et al., "The Potential of US Grazing Lands to Sequester Carbon and Mitigate the Greenhouse Effect," *Soil Science* 172, no. 12 (2007):943–56.

Mexico, and the cold windswept prairies of Canada. Then we'll know something about what works best in which places and under what conditions.

Planned rotational grazing is just one of many solutions that people are trying. Others include no-till farming, spreading microbially rich compost onto struggling grasslands, planting trees and other perennials in desertified areas, mixing charcoal ("biochar") into soil, where it creates living spaces for soil microorganisms, agroforestry (growing crops in a multistoried forest), silvopasturing (grazing animals in forests and orchards), and many, many other forms of management.

There will never be one right way to restore soil, because every place, every situation, is different. The Earth is not a machine. The Earth is a living system, powered by sunlight, constantly evolving and changing and breathing.

One thing we do know for sure is that by restoring soil with farming and grazing methods like the ones Peter and I are collecting data on, we can address a multitude of health-related concerns while we work toward drawing down CO_2 from the atmosphere: global water security, global hunger, failing local economies, issues of flooding, drought, and wildfires, conflicts over land and water, and pollution of rivers and lakes by runoff from large industrial farms, just to mention a few.

There is a phrase going around in my social circles these days: "The answer is soil. The question is irrelevant."

From Compost to Climate: A Hospital Changes Its Ways

Most hospital food is grown using extractive practices that are degrading topsoil and sending more CO_2 into the atmosphere. But what if hospitals could participate in *restorative* agriculture? What if hospital food became part of the movement to create healthier ecosystems in general?

"But I Thought Cows Were Bad for the Climate . . ."

Feedlot beef is one of the most fossil fuel–dependent foods we eat. For a single calorie of industrially farmed, grain-finished beef, farmers use 35–40 calories of fossil fuel energy to produce it, and that does not include transportation or processing.[*][†]

Yet 100 percent grass-fed beef, on properly managed land, is one of the *least* fuel-dependent foods we can eat. To produce one calorie of grass-fed beef uses no fuel: only a cow, standing in the sunshine, drinking out of a stream, munching on grass. The carbon footprint of that cow (or sheep or goat or caribou), if the land is managed properly to mimic natural grazing patterns, actually becomes a *negative* footprint, turning atmospheric CO_2 into living carbon in a multitude of forms.

Those fuel-efficient grass-fed calories also translate into an exceedingly nutrient-dense and therefore efficient form of calories for us. Arctic explorers and Inuit hunters lived for months at a time, with no adverse health effects, on nothing but "pemmican"—dried meat and fat from grazing animals mixed with a few berries—because it was the most dense and efficient food they could carry.[‡]

[*]   David Pimentel and Marcia Pimentel, "Sustainability of Meat-Based and Plant-Based Diets and the Environment," *American Journal of Clinical Nutrition* 78, no 3 Suppl (2003):660S–63S.

[†]   Leo Horrigan, Robert S. Lawrence, and Polly Walker, "How Sustainable Agriculture Can Address the Environmental and Human Health Harms of Industrial Agriculture," *Environmental Health Perspectives* 110, no. 5 (2002):445–56.

[‡]   Vilhjalmur Steffansen, "Adventures in Diet," *Harper's Magazine*, November 1935.

Back in 1992, Hollie Shaner, who worked in nutrition services at the University of Vermont Medical Center,[22] started a program to compost all of the hospital's cafeteria waste. This small but significant act was just hopeful enough that it inspired the staff and triggered a cascade of other green policies at the hospital, starting in the kitchen and eventually extending out into every other area.

UVM Medical Center is now one in a growing group of forward-thinking hospitals that have radically changed their relationship to food and farming. In 2007, the hospital initiated a three-year plan to phase out all industrially raised, antibiotic-fed animal products from the hospital food service. Now, more than 80 percent of the beef that is served there is local and grass fed, and 100 percent of the beef is free of nontherapeutic antibiotics. More than half of all the eggs and chicken they serve is organic.

Close to half of all the food prepared at the hospital is from local farms and local producers of cheese, breads, and grains. The vast majority of the food is also made to order. These policies reduce the hospital's impact on the environment, build resiliency against future price hikes of industrial food, and create strong relationships between the community of local farmers and the hospital. They also help patients and staff feel well cared for.

The hospital's relationship to food attracts new staff members. "Two medical residents this year said they chose to work here specifically because they were excited by what we were doing with food," says Diane Imrie, director of nutrition services at the hospital.

I asked Imrie how the local and organic foods project got started. She explained that she attended a retreat with Health Care Without Harm[23] at a time that she was having a "convergence of awareness" around three key issues: the impact of industrial food production

---

22 Formerly Fletcher Allen Hospital.
23 Health Care Without Harm, www.noharm.org, is an international coalition of hospitals and health-care systems, medical professionals, community groups, health-affected constituencies, labor unions, environmental and environmental health organizations, and religious groups working on environmentally responsible health care.

on climate change; the nation's "epidemic of obesity" related to poor nutrition and industrialized food; and the link between industrial meat and antibiotic-resistant infections, which they were struggling with at the hospital.

Since then, Imrie, who is also the coauthor of a cookbook called *Cooking Close to Home,* has initiated one project after another to move toward creating a hospital that serves nothing but local, organic, nutritious, and seasonally appropriate foods, with strong ties to local farmers and producers. She's not alone, but she is leading the charge.

As of 2015, more than 550 of the nation's 5,754 hospitals have signed Health Care Without Harm's "Healthy Food in Health Care Pledge." This means that they:

- Initiate on-site farmers' markets
- Act as pick-up sites for CSAs (Community Supported Agriculture projects)
- Plant food gardens
- Alter contracts with food distributors to eliminate packaged and canned foods
- Develop relationships with—and invest in—local farms
- Increase use of locally grown foods in their own hospital food services for patients, staff, and visitors[24]

One of the very first hospitals to sign the pledge was UVM Medical Center.

A Doctor Picks His First Tomato

The UVM Medical Center has three thriving gardens from which they harvest well over 400 pounds annually of herbs, lettuces, eggplant, tomatoes, peppers, and other vegetables, as well as blue-

---

24 "Healthy Food in Health Care: A Pledge for Fresh, Local, Sustainable Food," noharm. org, accessed September 27, 2012, http://www.noharm.org/lib/downloads/food/ Healthy_Food_in_Health_Care.pdf.

berries, kiwis, and limes. The largest garden, 75' x 30', is at their
rehab campus, where beehives provide honey for the hospital while
helping to pollinate the fruit and vegetable crops. A small but beautiful Healing Garden, created in memory of a patient, grows outside
the chemotherapy infusion bays.

The crowning glory is their rooftop garden, which sits on top of
the underground radiation oncology building and has rows of fruit
trees, a plum grove, herbs, and raised beds for vegetable production.
It also includes a children's tasting garden—where kids can sample
red runner beans, cherry tomatoes, nasturtiums, and herbs—as well
as a demonstration rainwater-capture unit on the toolshed. Signs
in the garden educate visitors about how rooftop gardens save air-
conditioning and heating costs, decrease the heat-island effect on
the surrounding environment, and mitigate storm-water runoff.

Imrie tells a story from the early days when she was doing all
the gardening work. She was going on vacation and asked a fellow
employee if he would mind picking the ripe tomatoes while she was
away. "It turned out he had never picked a tomato before. So I went
out there and showed him how to do it and let him taste all the
varieties. The funny thing is that now, several years later, you can
ask a team of people to go weed or pick vegetables and they just go
and do it. People who work here now think of it as a normal part of
a hospital workday."

Lisa Hoare now oversees all the gardens at UVM Medical Center
and tries to integrate permaculture principles wherever possible.
She explained to me that the rooftop garden eventually became a
teaching garden for staff—specifically staff that had absolutely no
gardening experience whatsoever—offering garden plots and free
weekly two-hour classes.

It was a huge success. Those staff members are now starting
gardens at home and are eager to mentor other staff members. "This
was a case," says Hoare, "where we had a choice between making a
very small impact on a lot of people [by using the garden to grow

a little extra food for the cafeteria, when local foods were already integrated into the supply chain] or making a very large impact on a few people—by giving staff members a life-changing learning experience that will continue to impact other people around them. I think we made the right choice."

A Culture Shift Among Staff

Food is just one area in which UVM Medical Center strives to be the greenest health-care organization in the country. One by one, staff have picked up on the passion for sustainability that the food services people started. Now the entire hospital is working on projects to reduce energy consumption, waste, and carbon outputs, as well as switching to environmentally friendly cleaning and lawn-care products.

The keys to the hospital's ongoing success are two employee-founded groups that spearhead initiatives. The "Green Team" meets regularly to gather ideas and set goals and then works with all departments to achieve them. A management-level "Sustainability Council" led by one of the hospital's vice presidents, with directors from most departments, works with the Green Team to prioritize and fund the projects.

Imrie says the hospital's success is due to several factors: the employees are very proactive and action oriented; the Sustainability Council has the authority to make decisions, which streamlines the initiatives; and there is strong support from the medical center's CEOs. "No one person has this job, it's everybody's job," Imrie explains, "and that is why it has been so effective. There are so many people working on these sorts of projects here, and it is such a normal part of the way we do things now, that when someone starts a major new initiative I often won't even get an email about it. It's no longer big news."

Keeping Drug Waste Out of the Water Supply

Typical of a hospital of its size, UVM Medical Center generates close to 60,000 pounds per year of drug waste. I asked John Berino, the hospital's director of environmental health and safety, what that means.

"Drug waste is just what the name says," he replied. "It includes 'spiked' IVs, pharmacy-prepared products, expired or discontinued medicines, pills, and full or partially full medicine vials and syringes."

Berino explained to me that the Environmental Protection Agency's regulations for drug waste date back to the 1970s and are shamefully outdated. "If we followed the outdated EPA regulations, less than one percent of this would actually be regulated and required to be disposed of as hazardous waste. The rest would be going down the drain into nearby Lake Champlain, or into the landfill via trash or red bag waste. This is detrimental to the environment and illegal in some cases, but that's what most hospitals are currently doing."

After nearly a year of multidisciplinary team meetings, the medical center enacted a system-wide drug waste collection and disposal process. Given the myriad conflicting regulations and the difficulty of separating out certain types of regulated drug wastes, they decided to adopt an approach that is simple and manageable: they now collect *all* drug waste. "While this represents a large change in our waste program, at added cost, it is certainly the best way for us to uphold our environmental mission," says Berino.

All of that waste is collected, handled, and disposed of using Best Available Control Technology (BACT). The waste is sent for high-temperature incineration at a fully regulated site, with one exception: their solvent waste is actually used, in part, to fuel the incinerators.

Reducing Footprints

UVM Medical Center reimburses its employees for using public transit and encourages carpooling by offering gas coupons and the best parking spots to carpoolers. Carpoolers are guaranteed a ride home from work if a transportation problem comes up—for example, a sick child is at home or the other carpoolers need to stay late. On a typical day, 300–400 of the medical center's employees carpool to work. Employees who bike or walk to work receive gift cards—worth a grand total of more than $77,000 since the program was initiated. Some of the staff members live in a nearby cohousing community and carpool or bike to work from there.

The hospital oversees thirty-five local patient care sites and 100 different outreach services throughout Vermont and upstate New York, making it easier for patients to get care close to home. The clinics themselves are being influenced by the hospital's commitment to sustainability. One clinic in particular, Milton Family Practice—where eight attending physicians and eighteen residents service 25,000 appointments per year—has taken on the goal of reaching a net-zero carbon footprint. When I last talked with them, they were in the process of installing solar panels that will provide 40 percent of the clinic's electricity. This is a significant amount of energy in an 11,500-square-foot building with twenty-two meeting and exam rooms, a radiography lab, an emergency/procedure room, and an X-ray lab—with computer equipment in every room.

Imrie says it is hard to convey the depth of what is going on at her hospital and the other hospitals, farms, and organizations that have gotten involved in serving local, grass-fed, and organic foods to their patients and staff, and working on energy conservation, as well. She especially likes the way they visit each other and get together for yearly retreats to share ideas. "We are like a team in Vermont and several surrounding states. Everyone is doing things in their own way, which is great, because we all get to learn from each other."

Make no mistake, UVM Medical Center is only in the first steps of its journey toward sustainability and resiliency. It is still a high-tech hospital with a large carbon footprint, but it gives us an idea of where we might start, and its efforts can feed our imagination as to where we might go.

Hospital as Community, Community as Hospital

Hospitals have the potential to be extraordinary places. What if all hospitals were *intentional* models of what fully functional, richly layered communities could look like, so that people came away from a hospital stay inspired to bring what they had experienced at the hospital back into their own lives?

Hospital stays could become more like retreats—oases where patients could focus on nothing but healing while their other basic needs, like food and shelter, were met. One could think of them as potential gathering places for top-notch healers to collaborate, working side by side and exchanging ideas, while also modeling for patients and their families how to live and work together in community.

Communities also have the potential to be healing places. A highly interconnected community can take on many roles that we typically look to a hospital to provide. If high-quality food, touch, company, and medical knowledge are free flowing within a community, if health-care providers live and work in each neighborhood, if there are safe spaces for people to rest and recuperate within a community, and if people take good care of their bodies, could modern hospitals, and their energy-intensive practices, become necessary for a much smaller number of cases?

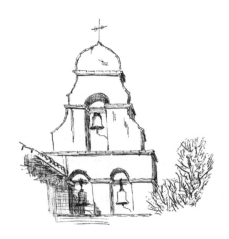

CHAPTER SEVEN

When the Machines Break and the Drugs Don't Arrive: The Need to Relocalize Care

"Strengthening health systems to enable them to deal with both gradual changes and sudden shocks is a fundamental priority in terms of addressing the direct and indirect effects of climate change for health."

—**World Health Organization, "Climate Change and Health"**

When the first oil crisis hit in 1973, I was ten years old. My brother and I sat in the backseat of our unheated station wagon getting bored and teasing each other while our single mother waited in line behind other frustrated drivers to buy gas. OPEC (a group of oil-exporting Middle Eastern countries) had put an embargo on the United States and several other countries for supplying arms to Israel. The price of oil quadrupled. Gas was rationed, with most stations closing (at President Nixon's request) from Saturday night until Monday morning. The era of "service stations" was over: gas stations stopped giving away steak knives and green stamps to try to entice customers to buy gas. Attendants stopped washing windows and waving at me and my brother, and they stopped offering to refill the oil or check the pressure in the tires as they pumped the gas. Instead, attendants rushed around with their heads down trying to stay out of the way of angry customers.

Hospitals, which were required to keep their thermostats at a minimum of 75 degrees, were hit hard by that oil crisis, as well as by the second oil crisis in 1979, when oil production dramatically dropped in Iran and Iraq due first to revolution and then to war. When, as a teenager, I went to work for my neurosurgeon grandfather, I didn't know that Hartford Hospital was struggling to pay its bills—spending *$10 a minute* just on heating the building on the coldest winter days. Fuel costs were $1.7 million for the year. When the hospital was designed in the 1960s, oil prices were a mere five cents a gallon, but by 1981 heating oil prices were a whopping $1.00 a gallon, twenty times higher than what they had planned for.[1] The oil crisis affected hospitals in other ways, as well. Plastic medical supplies like syringes were hard to obtain,[2] delayed in production because of shortages of petroleum—which is used as a raw material to make plastics, and as fuel to transport medical supplies from factories around the world to hospitals in places like Hartford, Connecticut.

Today's hospitals are far more dependent on fossil fuels than they were back then.

In the fall of 2007, the US went through a third oil crisis, but this time I wasn't sitting in the backseat punching my brother. This time I was the single mother driving the car, and I was the owner of the health-care facility, paying the bills.

The economic crisis unfolding around me was the first of several events that woke me up to the reality of the need to simplify and relocalize the way we care for each other during uncertain times.

By moving from my house into my clinic, I resolved some of my own dependency on fossil fuels, and by changing to a more communal business model, I solved some of my patients'—and my own—financial struggles. But every time I went to visit a patient in the hospital, and started to think on a larger scale, I felt uneasy again. It was one thing to convert my clinic into a more sustainable model. How in the world would a hospital do it, or an entire country's

1   Matthew L. Wald, "Hospitals Struggling to Contain Soaring Fuel Costs," *New York Times*, March 4, 1981.
2   Gary B. Clark and Burt Kline, "Impact of Oil Shortage on Plastic Medical Supplies," *Public Health Rep.* 96, no. 2 (1981):111–15.

health-care system? It seemed that in an era of increasing conflicts over oil rights, and increasing pressure to reduce our dependency on fossil fuels, hospital care could be dramatically impacted if there were a sudden price hike, another embargo, or simply a shortage of petroleum, as some people were predicting.

I had been to Cuba to research the amazingly successful way their health-care system responded to sudden oil shortages, but in the US we did not have the public-health infrastructure in place to make the transition as smoothly as they did. I wrote short articles about my concerns about the sustainability of our larger health-care system and posted them online.

One day a stranger named Dan Bednarz emailed me, saying, "We should talk."

Dan was a public-health professor who had recently gotten fired from his job at the University of Pittsburgh for insisting on talking about the end of cheap oil, and its impact on hospitals—an unpopular subject.

Dan combines an academician's love of statistics with a pessimist's view of the future. I can understand why people didn't really want to listen to him until after the economy fell apart and hurricanes Katrina, Irene, and Sandy hit. It's easy to discount wisdom that comes from the margins—where the people who have been pushed aside are often able to get a clearer view of the whole. Dan has a somber tone to his voice, perhaps from growing up in Detroit, where his father worked on an assembly line. But he was one of those truly astute people who, from his outpost, saw what was happening, and how it was happening—ahead of time—and was brave enough to talk about it, even if it meant losing his job.

He started a website called "Health after Oil" (https://health afteroil.wordpress.com/) and then found mine (www.sustainable medicine.org)—one of the only other websites discussing the same issues at that time. And he had learned, like I had, that it helps to make friends, especially when you've made a career out of proclaiming that the emperor has no clothes. Dan pointed me to the Post-

Carbon Institute and the Oil Drum, where other people were writing about climate change and the impact of rising oil prices on industrial agriculture, housing, and transportation, but very little about health care.

I suggested that we interview each other about our current thinking and concerns and then post the interviews online. Our interviews were like a perfect yin and yang outlook on the future of health care—he tackled gloomy looming problems, and I held out hopeful, idealistic solutions. Together we painted a relatively full picture of the conundrums and opportunities of transitioning to a health-care system that was more localized and less dependent on fossil fuels.

Those two interviews brought in emails from concerned medical students, people building clinics in Africa and India, radio hosts, and newspaper reporters. Soon I was appearing on panels discussing the future of health care, giving talks around the state, testifying at the statehouse, and meeting with hospitals. And Dan's online articles began getting *millions* of hits.

A Small New England Hospital's
Relationship to Petroleum

During a meeting with the "Green Team" of a small, independent New England hospital to discuss their fossil fuel use, I asked them to calculate how much the cost of oil would have to rise before they would no longer be a viable business. ·

Sitting around the table with upper management, a few providers, and the facilities manager, we calculated that if oil prices doubled, the cost of merely heating the building would eat up close to the entire amount that the hospital was currently clearing as profit. In other words, the hospital would just about break even—barely. Then I showed them a list I had compiled of all of the items in a hospital that are made of petroleum, and we started figuring in the costs of all the petroleum-based hospital supplies that would also double in price because they rely on oil for raw materials, production, and shipping.

It appeared likely that the hospital could go out of business in very short order if there were another embargo, or if oil prices suddenly rose. Being dependent on a single resource creates incredible instability in a system: if something goes wrong, it goes wrong in a very big way.

Our medical system is completely dependent on fossil fuels from side to side and from top to bottom, with the exception of a few wilderness first responders, herbalists, and hands-on healers who have never forgotten the basics. Our offices, our record keeping, our supplies, our tools, our diagnostic machines, our medicines, and our ambulances are all dependent on petroleum and other fossil fuels.

I showed the Green Team an article from the *Journal of the American Medical Association* that concurred: if there is an oil shortage due to another embargo, or if we successfully shift away from fossil fuels for the climate's sake, much of our current health-care system will need to be redesigned.[3]

The world's population is expected to increase from seven billion to eight billion between 2015 and 2030, and the US Department of Energy expects that unless we find entirely new sources of fuels by 2030, we will have about half the amount of oil and other liquid fuels that we had in 2011.[4] So that's all of us, plus one billion more people, to share half as much oil and other liquid fuels.

---

3   Howard Frumkin, Jeremy Hess, and Stephen Vidigni, "Peak Petroleum and Public Health," *JAMA* 298, no. 14 (2007):1688–90.
4   In April 2009, the United States Department of Energy held a round-table entitled "Meeting the Growing Demand for Liquid (fuels)." A graph in their presentation document shows that the Department of Energy expects a sharp decline of all known sources of liquid fuel supplies, starting in 2011. The graph, entitled "World Liquid Fuels Supply," drops from approximately 85 million barrels per day in 2011 to about half that by 2030. The graph contains a mysterious black line labeled "unidentified"— which represents as-of-yet-unknown sources of fuel that will be needed to fill the gap between rising demand and the decline of known supplies. (The already "identified" supplies include places where drilling has been put on hold due to environmental concerns). "Meeting the World's Demand: Liquid Fuels, A Roundtable Discussion," U.S Energy Information Administration, http://www.eia.gov/conference/2009/session3/Sweetnam.pdf.

Partial List of Health-Care Items Made out of Petroleum*

Supplies, including:
- Syringes
- IV bags
- Rubbing alcohol
- Bandages
- Antiseptics
- Oxygen tubing
- Thermometers
- Catheters
- Stethoscopes
- Sheets
- Pillows
- Blankets
- Beds
- Diapers
- Absorbent pads
- Bedpans
- Speculums
- Patient gowns
- Surgical masks
- Surgical gloves
- Surgical gowns
- Packaging for sterilizing equipment
- Disposable instruments
- Swabs
- Lancets
- Surgical tape
- Vaporizers
- Nebulizers

Most pharmaceutical drugs and other products, including:
- Anesthetics
- Antibiotics
- Antihistamines
- Cortisone
- Aspirin
- Antihistamines
- Cough syrup
- Antacids
- Glycerin
- Vitamins
- Lotions, ointments, salves
- Petroleum jelly
- Denture adhesives
- Laxatives
- Pill and medicine bottles
- Capsules
- Dispensing cups
- Eye-droppers
- Caps and lids

*   Sources: Illinois Oil and Gas Association, Ranken Energy Corporation, http://www.pbs.org/independentlens/classroom/wwo/petroleum.pdf.

Cleaning supplies, including:

- Disinfectants
- Ammonia
- Mops
- Sponges
- Buckets
- Soap
- Cleaning gloves
- Trash bags
- Biohazardous waste containers

Building materials, such as

- Linoleum floors
- Window casings
- Counters
- Storage units
- Paint
- Toilet seats
- Showers
- Shower curtains
- Equipment, such as:
- X-ray machines
- Ultrasound machines
- MRIs
- CT scanners
- PET scanners
- Radiological dyes

- Heart monitors
- Dental equipment
- Incubators
- Refrigerators and refrigerants

Office equipment and supplies, including:

- Electrical cords
- Lamps
- Telephones
- Computers
- Copiers
- Tape
- Pens
- Ink

Other important things, such as:

- Artificial limbs
- Artificial organs
- Heart valves
- Dentures
- Hearing Aids
- Eyeglasses

The upshot is this: by choice or by circumstance, we are going to have to find ways of providing health care that are not dependent on petroleum.

As I started telling this hospital's Green Team about very practical ways of creating resiliency in the workplace and lessening dependence on fossil fuels, I suddenly realized I had lost them.

Their eyes were glazed over. Their concern about a bleak future made it hard for them to pay attention to the alternatives I was about to propose. (That was when I understood how Dan Bednarz had lost his job: trying to explain these same issues to his colleagues.)

One of the biggest leadership challenges of this era is this: *how do we communicate urgency and relaxed confidence at the same time?* Clearly, in that meeting I did not succeed. As I try to get neighbors and colleagues to think about planning for the future, I've learned that I need to be able to hold up solutions at the same time that I explain the problems.

The small independent hospital I met with could have made changes that would have benefitted them and the community they served. If, like Muscogee Community Hospital in Oklahoma, they had invested in a geothermal heat pump, which uses the constant 55-degree temperature below the earth to draw in heat in the winter *and* cool in the summer, they could have recouped their investment relatively quickly through savings on heating oil and they would have been protected from one major aspect of fluctuating oil prices for decades to come (while reducing their carbon footprint at the same time). Instead, they waited and were bought by a larger hospital a few years later. This merger merely postpones the hospital's problem, because as we have learned, "too large to fail" is not an accurate assessment of any institution.

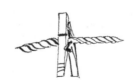

Technological Complexity Versus Natural Complexity: Which One Do We Want to Depend On?

Petroleum has allowed us to create an extremely complex society and an extremely complex medical system, with a huge amount of specialization, and innovation. Many good things have come out of this. But in order to maintain our medical system at this level of complexity we have to find ways of providing services that are unlikely to be affected by political upheavals, embargos, or the increasing pressure to reduce our impact on the climate. The technological complexity that fossil fuels have afforded us is too vulnerable, and too costly to our atmosphere, to continue to depend on for our entire health-care system.

I'd suggest that the complex systems we rely on for our health care from here on out should increasingly be the complexity of *natural systems*. We should be putting our time and money into the restoration of functionality of our soils, human relationships, microbiomes, and ecosystems.

The problem is not that we can't live without fossil fuels. The problem is that we have forgotten how. We have dismantled the landscapes that used to provide us with carbon-neutral food, fiber, and power. We live and work in skyscrapers that become useless during extended power outages, and in suburban neighborhoods that are hard to reach without vehicles. Most of us have forgotten how to travel without fossil fuels, how to build without them, and how to grow food without them. We have also forgotten how to take care of each other without them.

Like most people, I love many aspects of modern technology. I love being able to take photographs of my walks in the woods and send them instantly to my friends. I love being able to read obscure medical research online while sitting in front of the woodstove. I love the fact that a radiologist can show me exactly where my son Alden's collarbone has fractured (from doing stunts while sledding down the driveway), and predict how long it will take to heal. Yet in today's high-speed, competitive, petroleum-based world, vulnerability is not limited to the slender bones around our necks. As we do our daily stunts with our computers and cell phones and medical imaging machines, we are constantly sliding down the slippery slope of increasing dependence on modern technology in an era of increasing power outages, political upheavals, and supply-chain failures. And it is precisely our insistence on holding on to everything that creates the situation that threatens us with the very real possibility of losing everything.

Think about your mobile phone.

In a report by David Korowicz, called "Trade-Off: Financial System Supply-Chain Cross-Contagion, A Study in Global Systemic Collapse," he writes:

> Mobile devices, now ubiquitous, represent the culmination of twentieth-century physics, chemistry, and engineering. They signify thousands of direct—and billions of indirect—businesses and people who work to provide the parts for the phone, and the inputs needed for those parts, and the production lines that build them, the mining equipment for antimony in China, platinum from South Africa, and zinc from Peru, and the makers of that equipment.
>
> The mobile device [also] encompasses the critical infrastructures that those businesses require just to operate and trade—transport networks, electric grids and powerplants, refineries and pipelines, telecommunications and water networks—across the world. [The production of the mobile device] requires banks and stable money and the people and systems behind them. It requires a vast range of specialist skills and knowledge and the education systems behind them.[5]

5   David Korowicz, "Trade-Off: Financial System Supply-Chain Cross-Contagion: A Study in Global Systemic Collapse," research paper prepared for Metis Risk

If this is what is required to produce a cell phone, imagine then, what it takes to design, produce, and transport all the high-tech equipment used in a hospital. And imagine, then, how many things could go wrong in a war, a long-term power outage, or a natural disaster that prevents some part of the supply chain from operating smoothly.

A surgeon in a high-tech hospital—relying on machines with parts made around the globe, and disposable supplies—has a very high risk of being affected by events on the other side of the world. The risk lowers somewhat with each step toward simpler or more local technologies. A field surgeon trained to work in a tent with little equipment and few supplies is less likely to be affected than the surgeon who only has experience in a high-tech setting. An acupuncturist who uses needles, cotton balls, and alcohol has a small but still real risk of being affected. (I have to deal with needle shortages almost every time I place an order these days, but needles are a relatively simple technology that *could* be made locally if necessary, and can easily be resterilized using an autoclave.) An herbalist in South America who works with local herbs is *very* unlikely to be affected by a riot in Europe, a flood in China, or rising oil prices in the Middle East, because the supplies she needs grow right around her. Likewise, a lay midwife or massage therapist doesn't need much of anything except her own two hands. As we'll see in the upcoming chapters, a health-care system that figures out how to use public-health measures to support the creation of a healthy, resilient population can also maintain relative health and safety during emergencies.

As much as we might feel comforted by having the most advanced medical technology in the world, at times when natural and human-made disasters knock out power, topple factories, and disrupt supply chains both here and abroad, we may well find ourselves wishing for communities that are good at taking care of each other, and practitioners who are highly skilled in *low-tech* ways of preventing,

---

Consulting & Feasta, June 17, 2012, http://www.feasta.org/2012/06/17/trade-off-financial-system-supply-chain-cross-contagion-a-study-in-global-systemic-collapse/.

diagnosing, and treating illness. It is time to start creating those communities and educating ourselves in those low-tech skills.

Sudden shortages of certain medications and medical supplies have already started. Eighty-one percent of Canadian pharmacies reported that they were affected by drug shortages in 2010, partly due to a diminished supply of raw materials from China and India.[6] In the US, more than 90 percent of hematology/oncology pharmacists reported shortages in chemotherapy drugs in 2011. These shortages led to delays in chemotherapy, last-minute changes in the choice of therapies, complications in conducting clinical research, increases in the risks of medication errors and adverse outcomes, and increased medication costs for patients.[7]

In 2013, the Centers for Disease Control put out an emergency advisory that the United States was going through a shortage of doxycycline—the antibiotic of choice for treating Lyme disease and other insect-borne illnesses such as malaria, which are spreading northward due to climate change.[8] Tetracycline, also used for tick and other insect-borne diseases, was completely unavailable at the same time.[9, 10] The FDA also reported shortages in life-saving drugs, such as thyroid medication and epinephrine injections (epi-pens) for severe allergic reactions, as well as simple replacement minerals for IV bags, like sodium phosphate and sodium chloride.[11] An article in the *Washington Post* details

6   Canadian Pharmacists Association, Canadian Drug Shortages Survey Final Report, December 2010, http://www.pharmacists.ca/cpha-ca/assets/File/cpha-on-the-issues/DrugShortagesReport.pdf.
7   Ali McBride, et al., "National Survey on the Effect of Oncology Drug Shortages on Cancer Care," *American Journal of Health-System Pharmacy* 70, no. 7 (2013): 609–17.
8   "Nationwide Shortage of Doxycycline: Resources for Providers and Recommendations for Patient Care," Centers for Disease Control and Prevention, last updated June 12, 2013, accessed June 9, 2015, http://emergency.cdc.gov/HAN/han00349.asp.
9   Centers for Disease Control and Prevention, Doxycycline Shortage, last updated July, 31, 2014, accessed June 9, 2015, http://www.cdc.gov/std/treatment/doxycyclineShortage.htm.
10 http://www.fda.gov/Drugs/DrugSafety/DrugShortages/ucm314743.htm#tetracycline.
11 http://www.fda.gov/Drugs/DrugSafety/DrugShortages/ucm314743.htm#sodiumchloride.

shortages in intravenous nutrition for premature babies that are affecting the health and survival of babies in the United States far more than anywhere else. Sometimes, even though the supplies are available, in a for-profit system, once a company's patent has ended there is little motivation to continue manufacturing.[12] In six years, from 2006 to 2012, drug shortages in the United States skyrocketed from 70 drugs to 299 drugs, so much so that the FDA started a task force to look for solutions.[13]

Just-in-Time Inventories Might Be Too Late

According to Al Cook, a member of the Medical Materials Coordinating Group that advises the US Department of Health and Human Resources on emergency preparedness, many hospitals and manufacturers of hospital goods have switched to a "just-in-time" inventory system, meaning that they don't order new supplies, such as syringes, catheters, manufacturing materials, and food, until the supplies are depleted.[14] They do this with confidence, knowing that under normal circumstances, deliveries can happen within hours. This inventory system is considered essential for corporate competitiveness in a for-profit health-care system like ours. But it leaves hospitals, nursing homes, and pharmacies very vulnerable. If deliveries are stopped in an area due to a natural disaster or sudden fuel shortage, patient care is jeopardized.

Cook notes that there are not enough supplies in any local area to support the care necessary during a large-scale emergency.[15] This became painfully evident after Hurricane Katrina, when trucks

---

12 Alexandra Robbins, "Children Are Dying," *Washingtonian*, May 2, 2013, accessed June 9, 2015, http://www.washingtonian.com/articles/people/children-are-dying /index.php.
13 American Society of Health System Pharmacists, letter to FDA regarding FDA-2013-N-0124; Food and Drug Administration Drug Shortages Task Force and Strategic Plan, March 14, 2013.
14 Richard D. Holcomb, "When Trucks Stop, America Stops," American Trucking Association (paper prepared for the American Trucking Association, July 14, 2006).
15 Ibid.

loaded with emergency goods were rerouted, creating lengthy delays in deliveries of food and medical supplies to hospitals and residents in New Orleans.[16]

Richard Holcomb created a timeline outlining the potential consequences of restricting or halting truck traffic in response to a national or regional emergency in the United States.[17] The timeline illustrated that *within twenty-four hours*:

- Delivery of medical supplies to affected areas ceases.
- Hospitals run out of basic supplies, such as syringes and catheters, within hours.
- Radiopharmaceuticals for cancer treatment and diagnostics, which have an effective life of only a few hours, deteriorate and become unusable.
- Gas stations begin to run out of fuel.
- Medical and pharmaceutical manufacturers using "just-in-time" manufacturing develop shortages of raw materials and other components.
- US mail and other package delivery ceases.
- Food shortages begin to develop in hospitals, nursing homes, and supermarkets.

All this in just the first day. Within a week of the same scenario, hospitals will begin to exhaust oxygen supplies. Within two weeks the nation's clean water will begin to run dry, lacking the chemicals needed for water purification at water treatment facilities.

This report only deals with the effects of restricted trucking. Supply chains are also dependent on shipping by air, sea, and rail. The daily operations of our medical system are entirely dependent

16 Sheri Fink, *Five Days at Memorial: Life and Death in a Storm Ravaged Hospital* (London: Atlantic, 2013).
17 Richard D. Holcomb, "When Trucks Stop, America Stops," American Trucking Association (paper prepared for the American Trucking Association, July 14, 2006), accessed September 27, 2012, http://www.trucking.org/Newsroom/Trucks%20 Are/When%20Trucks%20Stop%20America%20Stops.pdf.

on fossil fuels, stable transport routes, and fair weather, both political and environmental.

Rethinking Disposability

When I went to acupuncture school in the early 1990s, we were still sterilizing needles and reusing them. By the time I graduated, four years later, nearly everyone was using needles that were chemically sterilized and packaged in plastic (i.e., petroleum), and we disposed of them after a single use. Awareness of AIDS, hepatitis C, and other blood-borne illnesses made a booming business out of disposable medical products in the 1990s, and I arrived on the scene just at that turning point. In all of health care, disposable plastics—for syringes, bags, tubing, surgical supplies, pill bottles, and bandages—have replaced reusable metal and glass, and in many areas disposable paper has replaced cloth items. Meanwhile we have forgotten we have other options, and most manufacturers have stopped making them.

Climate change, flooding, drought, fossil fuel shortages, and conflicts over water and other resources all act as destabilizing influences on political systems and economies. Local and national economies are increasingly intertwined with those of other countries. We rely on each other, around the world, for the technology, food, and other products we have become accustomed to. When one part of the world is affected, we are all affected. The question is, will we respond to shortages with mutual aid, cooperation, and collaboration, or with conflict? Can we learn to take care of each other in ways that rely on local supplies, natural processes, and simpler technologies? Can we invest in local manufacturers of essential drugs and medical supplies and ask our hospitals to return to using older methods of resterilizing supplies?

Perhaps we can learn to hold on to technology lightly: "Wow, it's really nice to have disposable plastic syringes and tubing, but I don't want the hospital to be entirely dependent on them because if

Dogs as Diagnosticians

Sophisticated diagnostic methods don't need to be expensive.
The most sophisticated piece of medical technology ever created
might be over in the corner of your kitchen, licking leftovers off
of your plate.

There are medical-alert dogs working with patients that can
tell when a person with diabetes is about to have a blood sugar
crisis, or when a person with narcolepsy is about to fall asleep,
or a person with epilepsy is about to have a seizure. In three
weeks you can train a dog to detect cancer with astonishing accu-
racy. "We are only at the start of working out everything dogs
can detect," the UK's *Daily Mail* quotes researcher Dr. Claire
Guest. "It would seem that almost any medical event has an odor
change. The clever thing is that the dogs are able to work out
what the norm is, and when it changes."[*]

A recent article about canine detection in the *New Yorker*
points to the superiority of dogs' noses over technology. "In the
1970s, researchers found that dogs could detect even a few particles per million of a substance; in the 1990s, more subtle instruments lowered the threshold to particles per billion; the most
recent tests have brought it down to particles per trillion."

Paul Waggoner, a behavioral scientist at the Canine Detection
Research Institute, at Auburn University, in Alabama, told the
reporter. "It's a little disheartening, really. I spent a good six
years of my life chasing this idea, only to find that it was all about
the limitations of my equipment."[†]

One Labrador, for instance, was 98 percent as accurate as a
colonoscopy when smelling stool samples, and 95 percent as
accurate when smelling breath samples. But it gets better than

---

[*]   Jenny Stocks, "The Dogs That Can Detect Cancer: Meet The 4-Legged Bio
      Detectives Who Are Pioneering a Health Revolution," *Daily Mail*, September
      13, 2012.
[†]   Burkhard Bilger, "Beware of the Dogs," *New Yorker*, February 27, 2012.

that—because the dog could also differentiate polyps from malignancies, which a colonoscopy cannot. In addition, the dog was especially accurate at finding early-stage cancers, which are very hard to detect with standard tests, but which, if they can be found, greatly increase the patient's chance of survival because they are easier to treat than late-stage cancers.[*]

"Detection of early-stage cancers is the real holy grail in bowel cancer diagnosis because surgery can cure up to ninety percent of patients who present with early-stage disease," said Trevor Lockett, a bowel cancer researcher in Australia.[†]

Colonoscopies are highly invasive tests, they cost from $2,000 to $3,000, they require anesthesia, and they have some serious risks. When polyp-like masses are found by colonoscopy, they are snipped out of the intestines and then need to be examined (at more expense) in a laboratory to see if they are malignant. Colonoscopies are also dependent on disposable supplies, high-tech equipment, and a functioning power grid. So why are we still using colonoscopies when we know that dogs can be trained to communicate diagnoses that are nearly as accurate and even more precise than a colonoscopy? Well, it turns out that dogs' noses are poking around in areas where they really are not welcome.

In article after article about cancer-sniffing dogs, not a single article concludes that we should simply train more dogs to do this, and work with them side by side. Instead, the articles conclude that cancer-sniffing dogs will be useful to develop technology that can screen for the odors the dogs are detecting. In other words: figure out how the dog does it, then create a technology that mimics it and can be patented, and put that into use to generate profits in a way that a dog cannot.

[*]   Eva Schaper, "Cancer Sniffing Dogs May Lead to Less Invasive Tests for Tumors," *Bloomberg*, February 1, 2011.
[†]   Ibid.

the supply truck can't get through, they won't have any other way to treat patients. So let's figure out what else might work, and then only use plastic when absolutely necessary."

Or, "I'm going to invest in this company making biomarker tests for cancer, but I'll take some of the money I make and put it toward a medical diagnostics dog-training site so that if manufacturing supplies run low, patients will have other options."

Or, "It's been great having the option of taking pain medication, but I would rather not be dependent on it, because if the manufacturer goes out of business, or there is a flood and the road washes out on the day I was supposed to pick up my prescription, I want to have other tools at my disposal that I can access no matter where I am. So I'm going to take this natural pain management course, eat foods that reduce inflammation, and go to a support group instead."

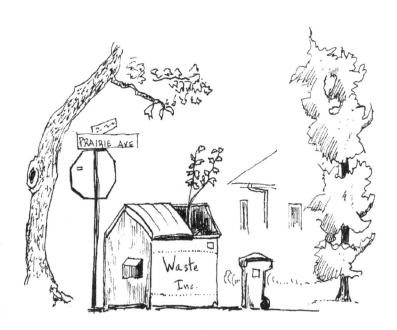

A Town Starts Planning to Relocalize Care

Some towns are doing health-care resiliency planning far in advance of any emergency. Sarah Edwards contacted me a couple of years ago looking for a consultation. Sarah is an ecopsychologist and prolific writer who also runs continuing education programs for mental health professionals who want to help people deal with the emotional ups and downs of a climate-challenged world. But that's not what she wanted help with. She wanted me to help her figure out what to do with her town.

She lives in a town of about 2,400 residents in California, far away from any health-care services, surrounded on four sides by the Los Padres National Forest. Their goal as a town is to be relatively independent in case their ability to access services is interrupted in the future. She knew that, with a changing climate, weather problems were on their way and, as a report from the town indicates, they are already being affected by rising oil prices and economic stresses. Sarah's report outlines her town's story.

> Pine Mountain Club was developed in the 1970s as a seasonal resort and quickly attracted couples who bought lots and built second homes with plans to retire here, which many did. We still have a significant contingent of retired residents, many of whom are living on fixed incomes. But with our lack of health services, the later years of retirement become a challenge, and many moved back to an urban area in time. We are now home to a diverse population that includes professional pre-retirees and young families with small and teen-aged children who have fled the city for lower housing costs and a safer, healthier way of life. Approximately 2,000 additional residents are "weekenders" or "holiday-only" property owners, who come in from other areas to relax and recreate.

All well and good . . . idyllic almost . . . until one
confronts the drastically changing state and national
economy and the very real prospect of a future when
traveling a considerable distance for jobs and nearly all
basic services becomes a costly challenge.

Throughout the town's history, most people who had jobs
commuted an hour or more to get to their workplace. Everyone
commuted at least an hour for groceries, entertainment, and
health care. The Pine Mountain Club residents both earned and
spent nearly all their income elsewhere. In an age of cheap, abundant oil and fair California weather, this was never viewed as a
problem.

We were an idyllic nearby-faraway place. But like many
small rural communities and those on the far fringes of
metropolitan areas that grew when home prices were
soaring, we're being hit hard by a dramatically shifting
economy.
    Property values have fallen 47 percent, and we're
suffering a high number of foreclosures. Thus the
collapse of the real estate market has left many older
residents who would have moved to be closer to health
services unable to sell their homes, and "stranded" in
our community. At the same time, energy costs have
risen significantly in California, making trips to the
city run at least $50 per trip. Small businesses here,
of which there are few, are closing or struggling. We
have the highest vacant-home rate (61 percent) and the
highest percent of people whose incomes are below the
poverty level (17 percent) in the area, nearly double that
of what are considered "poorer" nearby communities.
The California Employment Development Department

reports our unemployment rate as of February 2009 to
be 15.4 percent. This is higher than the 13.8 percent rate
in Kern County and the 11.4 percent rate for California
as a whole.

An out-of-sight, out-of-mind stepchild, "at the end
of the line," in the far southwest corner of resource-
strapped Kern County, we are underserved in terms of
public services. Essentially we're a community without a
safety net, something few expected we would need, but
which we must now build.

In 2005, inspired by the Post Carbon Institute and the US
Transition Town Movement, an informal group of volunteers started
a nonprofit called Let's Live Local. The group was concerned about
the effects of rising oil prices, climate change, and resource deple-
tion on their community and the surrounding national forest. They
set out to identify the steps they would need to take (given their
small size and remote location) to develop access to local food and
energy and to be able to live, shop, and work locally. They decided
that one of the most crucial services they needed to develop locally
was health care.

Over a period of several months, Sarah and I talked about many
strategies for relocalizing health care. The town did an inventory of
health-care needs—including the townspeople's medications—and
set out to find a doctor willing to live there. First, the community
found a "house call" doctor who purchased a weekend home and
was willing to practice there one weekend a month. Then, with his
help, they started the search for a doctor willing to live and practice
there year-round. They trained six Family Care Giving Practitioners
through the Red Cross and established a referral network with one
toll-free number so residents could reach out directly to caregivers,
the house-call doctor, a coalition of mental health workers, and
other resources.

An herbalist moved to town, and they worked with her to come up with alternatives to medications. They started asking residents to be sure to have several months' worth of extra medication on hand in case there was an interruption in supplies due to a forest fire or other disaster. In addition, residents started a community garden and many home gardens, for growing food and medicinal herbs.

Let's Live Local also started three cooperative businesses: a beef coop with a local rancher, an organic produce coop with a regional community-supported agriculture project, and a wood pellet coop helping more than 150 families heat their homes using a renewable resource.

In 2014, after much work, the town finally was able to open a clinic. They have more to do before they are truly resilient, but unlike many small towns in similar circumstances, most residents there now know what they are facing, and what needs to be done.

As we transition into a post-petroleum and climate-challenged world, we can include our neighbors in our planning, and be both safer and stronger because of our collaboration. Building resiliency means strengthening our relationships and investing in community and collective skills for the future.

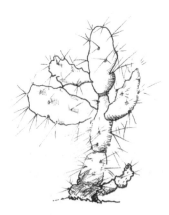

CHAPTER EIGHT

Cuba's Experiment in Post-Petroleum Health Care

"Medicine is a social science, and politics nothing but medicine
on a grand scale."
—**Rudolph Virchow**

I t looks kind of rusty here," said my four-year-old son Henry, clutching his toy tiger, when he woke up and looked out the window on his first day of our travels.

He was right. Cuba was kind of rusty. The cars were very old, the paint on the buildings was peeling, and the roads were full of potholes. It was 1999, and this small country had been in a crisis for about a decade, ever since shifting politics on the other side of the globe cut the country off from its main source of petroleum, almost overnight.

Cuba had depended on the Soviet Union for most of their trade, in large part because the US embargo had prevented Cuba from importing goods from its closest neighbor since 1960. When the Soviet bloc collapsed in the late 1980s, Cuba was suddenly stranded with almost no access to petroleum and other supplies they had come to depend on. The economy suffered; they lost 85 percent of their trade. Food, basic medicines, and medical supplies—already in short supply due to the embargo—became even more scarce. Farms lost the fertilizers and pesticides used for industrial agriculture. Fuel shortages made it hard to transport people and goods even a few miles, and blackouts lasted as long as sixteen hours a day. And the island happened to be in the hurricane belt, as well.

This crisis, which Cuba ironically dubbed "the Special Period," was like a trial run through many of the energy-descent and climate-related scenarios that are now affecting communities worldwide.

In most countries, during stressful times like these, serious conflicts arise, and people's health deteriorates as they struggle to adapt. Cubans, however, turned this crisis into an opportunity. Through innovation and sharing, they transformed both their medical and agricultural systems in creative ways that actually *improved* the health of their own citizens. An already strong interest in preventive, community, and alternative medicine blossomed, as much of the oil-dependent high-tech medicine became impossible to provide. During that same period, they started a free international medical school, treated millions of patients for free around the world, and invented several groundbreaking drugs.

Long before I was thinking about my personal relationship to fossil fuels, sustainability, or climate, but curious to see one of the world's most successful health-care experiments, I traveled to Cuba to study the creative ways their medical system was responding to the limited material resources of the Special Period. Being relatively at ease in Spanish, I chose not to go with an organized tour, preferring to poke around by myself and see if I could figure out what was really going on. I traveled (with US State Department approval for research) on my own itinerary, which unfolded from one conversation to the next. Looking back, I'm quite sure that my unbending faith that we can face our current challenges with an innovative spirit and come out stronger is due in large part to what I saw there.

Adapting to the Special Period

When the Soviet supply chain vanished, food quality and people's caloric intake in Cuba dropped dramatically at first. People woke up to the reality that, other than fish and sugarcane, they didn't have much of a local food system. Cuba reserved most of their fresh seafood for the restaurants in coastal areas (where Europeans flock to the gorgeous beaches), in a desperate attempt to bring cash into the country. Cheap and often donated staples, such as rice, beans, and canned meat, kept people alive. During parts of my visit, nearly every meal included hot dogs—donated by some generous country. (My son Henry, of course, was delighted.)

City neighborhoods quickly started planting community gardens, fruit trees, rooftop gardens, and even troughs along the sidewalks in which to grow vegetables so they wouldn't have to use the precious remaining gas supplies to truck food in from the countryside. The Cuban government rationed food to make sure everyone had some, while they worked to convert their huge mono-cropped farming cooperatives of sugarcane and tobacco—grown for export—into smaller, multifaceted organic farms growing vegetables, meat, eggs, and fruit to feed their own people. Farm animals worked, while tractors sat idle.

Picking up hitchhikers became mandatory, to conserve the little fuel that was left. Anything that could be used for public transport, was. Even dump trucks became buses: after dropping off materials, they shuttled people to work and children to school.

As the amount of hard currency available for medicine and medical technology shrank, the strength of the Cuban public-health system was put to the test. Amazingly, although food was scarce, the health of their citizens, which was already excellent, continued to improve between 1990 and 2000, their most difficult decade.

In 1990, at the beginning of the Special Period, Cuba's infant mortality rate was 10.7 infant deaths per 1,000 live births. By 1995, it had improved slightly, to 9.4, and by 2000 it had improved even more dramatically to 7.2. Since then, things have gotten even better, with infant mortality rates in Cuba dropping to 4.7 in 2014

Is Cuba Lying?

Some critics of Cuba have suggested that their figures are falsified in order to glorify their political system. An article in the *International Journal of Epidemiology*[*] makes a powerful argument for this being nearly impossible, due to the high degree of detail that Cuba provides on all their statistics. No pregnancy, illness, or death ever goes unnoticed by the Ministry of Public Health because every single Cuban has a nurse-and-doctor team living right in their immediate neighborhood whose only job is to improve and track the health of those living around them. This detailed accounting is, in many ways, the essence of their family-doctor system and its resulting public-health success.

[*]   Richard S. Cooper, et al., "Health in Cuba," *International Journal of Epidemiology* 35, no. 4 (2006):817–24.

(better than the 6.17 in the US and, astonishingly, better than the global average of 34).[1]

Mortality rates of children under age five showed the same pattern of improvement: 13.2 in 1990, 12.5 in 1995, and 11.1 by 2000. Only life expectancy dipped slightly during the worst years: 75.2 in 1989, 74.8 in 1995, then back up to 76 by 2000, and 78.2 by 2014.[2,3]

---

1   Central Intelligence Agency, "World Factbook," accessed September 27, 2012, https://www.cia.gov/library/publications/the-world-factbook/.
2   Annual Statistical Yearbook, Ministry of Public Health, Havana, 2003, and CIA World Factbook.
3   Just to compare: in the US, infant mortality rate was 9.8 in 1989 and 7 in 2000; life expectancy in the US was 75.1 in 1989 and 76.7 in 2000.

Overall, the health, life expectancy, and infant mortality and survival rates of Cubans are very similar to those of people in the United States. So here's the big difference: in the United States we spend more than $9,500[4,5] per person, per year, on health care (more money than any other country, and more of our GDP—nearly 18 percent), while Cubans spend roughly $400 (and only 10 percent of their GDP) to get similar results.[6,7]

It's probably not the diet of donated hot dogs. How does Cuba keep its citizens healthy on such a small budget, with so many economic challenges?

More importantly, *what can we learn from them?*

Embedded Care: The Family Doctor Program

At the time the supply-chain crisis hit, everything in Cuba's health-care system was already set up to work for the common good: similar to the way our roads, water, fire, police, and elementary school systems are set up in the United States. Cuba's public infrastructure includes medical schools, community clinics, hospitals, and pharmaceutical research labs and manufacturers. All of these are supported by common funds and provide health care, medical training, and medicines free of charge to the public. This free, centralized health-care system also allows them to try out and track the success of new ideas for care.

---

4   Centers for Medicare and Medicaid, National Health Expenditures 2014 Highlights, http://www.cms.gov/Research-Statistics-Data-and-Systems/Statistics-Trends-and-Reports/NationalHealthExpendData/Downloads/highlights.pdf.
5   World Health Organization, Global Health Observatory database, accessed November 2, 2014, www.who.int/gho/countries/usa/en/.
6   World Health Organization Global Health Observatory database, accessed November 2, 2014, www.who.int/gho/countries/cub/en/ 2012 data.
7   Cuba is not alone. Other regions, like Sri Lanka, China, and the state of Kerala in India, are also known as "low-income, high well-being" areas, especially when it comes to health. The UC Atlas of Global Inequality, Health Care Spending, accessed June 9, 2015, http://ucatlas.ucsc.edu/spend.php.

In the mid-1980s, just a few years before the Special Period, Cuba started a pilot program embedding primary care physicians in one neighborhood in Havana, to see if it would improve the health of those who lived there. The pilot was so successful that the Ministry of Public Health quickly expanded its goal toward putting a primary care doctor-nurse team in all neighborhoods. By the 1990s Cuba had reached its goal. Every neighborhood in the country now has its own family physician and nurse team, providing care for 120–160 families.[8]

By living in the same neighborhood where they work, these doctor-nurse teams are on call for acute problems, can teach and practice preventive care to whole families, can notice issues while patients are going about their daily lives, and can easily make house calls. This sort of regular contact—both casual and professional— lessens the need for emergency room visits, hospital stays, and nursing homes, and gives the teams a rich, multilayered understanding of each patient's whole situation, allowing them to intervene long before most doctors would notice a problem brewing. Even when a family seems healthy, the teams make an annual visit to every citizen's home to look for potential issues—such as places where elders might trip and fall, or signs that a child is being neglected—that might need intervention.[9]

With such easy access to primary care, Cubans are less likely to postpone diagnostic tests or put off a visit to a doctor. Illnesses are caught and treated sooner, and, in the case of contagious illness, are less likely to spread. Neighborhood doctors and nurses are part of the team when someone is hospitalized, and they are there to take over when patients are discharged from the hospital.

The teams aren't just providing medical care. They also do public-health studies to identify trends of illness, assess environmental and

8   J. M. Feinsilver, *Healing the Masses: Cuban Health Politics at Home and Abroad* (Berkeley: University of California Press, 1993).
9   Christina Perez, *Caring for Them from Birth to Death* (Lanham: Rowman & Littlefield Publishers, 2008).

social problems, and set priorities for treatment of epidemic diseases and upcoming prevention campaigns.[10] There is also an aspect of community activism in their work: Because these providers are raising their own families in the same neighborhoods where they see patients, they have extra motivation to create safe, healthy neighborhoods. In this embedded role, they can engage with the people around them to reduce drug use, teach about healthy relationships, and clean up problems like broken glass or sewage leaks.

"Polyclinics," spread throughout the country, are hubs for the Family Doctor Program, with each polyclinic serving from twenty to forty neighborhoods. By arranging health care in evenly spaced concentric circles (rather than allowing providers to congregate in wealthy urban areas or nicer neighborhoods while avoiding low-income areas), everyone in the country is guaranteed relatively equal access to care. The polyclinics serve as meeting spaces for family doctors and nurses to discuss cases with each other and with specialists, and as medical centers for patients to receive services and diagnostics that are not available in the local clinics. This allows family doctors to share the use of laboratories and expensive diagnostic equipment, as well—and ensures that all family doctors across the country have access to similar infrastructure, no matter where they practice.[11]

Cuba's investment in primary care, rather than in specialists, became a crucial advantage during the petroleum crisis in the 1990s. The primary care doctors adapted more easily to the lack of fuel and supplies, while the specialists, trained to rely heavily on technology, had a harder time continuing to care for patients. Specialists are particularly vulnerable to the kinds of challenges that oil shortages and economic collapse present.

Jomo Uduman notes that the collapse of socialist Europe and the

---

10 C. William Keck and Gail A. Reed, "The Curious Case of Cuba," *American Journal of Public Health* 102, no. 8 (2012):e13–e22.

11 Gail Reed, "Cuba's Primary Health Care Revolution: 30 Years On," *Bulletin of the World Health Organization* 86, no. 5 (2008):321–416.

The HIV/AIDS Crisis in Cuba

Changes and revisions in Cuba's health-care system are frequent. Some changes are top-down and proactive: When AIDS appeared on the international horizon, Cuba's Ministry of Public Health was all over it. The ministry instituted many successful policies to quell the HIV/AIDS epidemic, such as regular testing of the entire population, early access to prenatal care, and early treatment for mothers and children with HIV.

The *New York Times* attributed Cuba's rapid and effective response to the HIV/AIDS crisis to the fact that their leader, Fidel Castro, is a voracious reader and has "high beams" focused on worldwide health issues.*

But changes in Cuba's health-care system also come from grass roots upwards. In any experimental system, mistakes are part of the learning process, and feedback has to be

---

*   Donald G. McNeil Jr., "A Regime's Tight Grip on AIDS," *New York Times*, May 7, 2012.

---

tightened US embargo on Cuba did not affect all levels of Cuba's public health system equally. "The greater the specialization, the greater the harm that was done. This is true, of course, because more specialized treatments require sophisticated and expensive equipment, disposable parts, and other supplies."[12]

The majority of doctors in the United States are specialists, not primary care doctors.

---

12 Jomo Uduman, "The Cuban Approach to Health Care: Origins, Results, and Current Challenges Evolution in the Revolutionary Period," *Colombo Herald*, October 19, 2010.

incorporated into the next phase of the experiment. Some early policies, although "successful," were quite unpopular—such as quarantining everyone with AIDS to prevent the spread of the HIV virus. AIDS patients and their families were dissatisfied with the policy that all people with AIDS were required to live in a sanitorium, so those families, along with many physicians, lobbied the Ministry of Public Health until the quarantine policy was finally changed.*

The end result of Cuba's proactive—and evolving—strategies is that Cuba has a dramatically lower incidence of HIV (0.1 percent) than most other countries.[†] In 2013, only two children in Cuba were born with HIV. In 2015, the World Health Organization declared that Cuba was the first country to eliminate the transmission of HIV (and syphilis) from mother to child.

*   Ibid.
†   C. William Keck and Gail A. Reed., "The Curious Case of Cuba," *American Journal of Public Health* 102, no. 8 (2012):e13–e22.

Duct Tape on the X-ray Machines

"We could live the rest of our lives on the garbage from your country," said my host, Elena, as she sat cutting up her daughter's old math homework into squares to be used as toilet paper. "We would repair all those computers and clothes you throw away." Her voice carried a sense of pride in her country's ability to resuscitate things.

Most people have seen the photos: the streets in Cuba are like a movie set from the 1950s—full of beautiful old cars Cubans have kept running since the embargo started. But the cars are just the tip of the iceberg of the Cubans' ability to make things last. When I was traveling in Cuba, my eyeglasses broke and I lost the screw that was needed to put them back together. I saw a man sitting and repairing watches at a small table on a sidewalk, and asked him if he had a screw that would work. He did not, but instead he took the glasses from me, and using a small piece of wire from an unfolded paperclip, some nail clippers, and a little hammer, he proceeded to fashion a tiny rivet that not only worked perfectly, but would never fall apart again. It only took about fifteen minutes, because he had the skills to do it using everyday items that all of us have at home.

The health-care workers were just as resourceful. At one hospital I visited, the X-ray machine was held together with duct tape but still worked fine. A homeopathic pharmacy was fashioning little dispensing envelopes out of folded paper, since they didn't have any bottles, or even any tape to hold the paper envelopes closed.

Knowing that Cubans were literally holding things together with shoestrings, I had brought some things with me to donate and felt conflicted as to which of the many clinics I visited I should give them to. But as I dropped off a bunch of books and medical journals at one clinic, the acupuncturist there told me not to worry: after he read them, he would pass them along to the next clinic, and they would keep circulating from one clinic to the next, until eventually they landed in a central lending library for health-care providers. This was standard practice whenever new reading materials arrived.

Sharing also happened on a national level. When money for supplies became scarce, the Minister of Public Health initiated a Tuesday morning meeting of all major health sectors to assess the exact amount of hard currency available that week, and to decide which medications and equipment to spend it on. Cuban hospitals did the same, meeting once a week to tally the medications on hand and send out requests to neighboring hospitals and pharmacies to find and share medications for patients whose needs couldn't be met locally.[13] The focus was on saving lives.

13 Jomo Uduman, "The Cuban Approach to Health Care: Origins, Results, and Current Challenges Evolution in the Revolutionary Period," *Colombo Herald*, October 19, 2010.

A United Nations report from 1999 stated that "Cuba is the country with the best health situation in Latin America and the Caribbean. It is also the country that has achieved the most effective impact with resources, although scarce, invested in the health sector."[14]

Revolutionary Medicine

Cuba's system of free medical care was basically built from scratch.

In 1959, just before the Cuban Revolution, there were only 6,300 physicians, two-thirds of whom lived in the capital city of Havana. There was only one rural hospital in the entire country. In the decade following the revolution, nearly half of those physicians left the country, leaving only sixteen professors at Cuba's sole medical school, and only one doctor for every 2,500 citizens.[15,16,17]

In 1960, a year after the revolution, Doctor Ernesto "Che" Guevara gave a speech called "On Revolutionary Medicine" in which he noted how the wealthy class background of the remaining doctors was preventing them from seeing the necessity of helping poor rural patients without being given special pay for the hardship of living under harsh conditions:[18]

> A few months ago, here in Havana, it happened that a group of newly graduated doctors did not want to go into the country's rural areas, and demanded remuner-

14 United Nations Development Programme, *Study on Human Development and Equity in Cuba* (New York: Oxford University Press, 1999), 103.

15 C. William Keck and Gail A. Reed., "The Curious Case of Cuba," *American Journal of Public Health* 102, no. 8 (2012):e13–e22.

16 E. L. Baker and Cuba Study Group, *The Cuban Health Care System and Its Achievement. Cuba's Health System: an alternative approach to health delivery* (Houston: University of Texas Health Science Center at Houston, 1975).

17 Centro Nacional de Información de Ciencias Médicas, *Emigración Médica* (1968), 21–26.

18 See the film *Salud* for an interesting re-visit of this scenario in Venezuela.

ation before they would agree to go. From the point of view of the past it is the most logical thing in the world for this to occur; at least, so it seems to me, for I can understand it perfectly . . .

Guevara spoke from experience. He himself was from a wealthy Argentinean family, part Irish, part Basque, and part Spanish, and grew up reading everyone from Robert Frost to Albert Camus and Karl Marx. While in medical school, however, he and a biochemist friend took a now-famous motorcycle ride throughout South America, which gave him a view into the lives and health problems of the rural poor in deeply divided class societies. This gave him a new mission to change society through medical care itself, which ultimately brought him to Cuba.[19] Health care and education were at the forefront of his ideas of revolution. In the speech, he goes on to talk about the need to develop a medical school that would train the rural poor themselves as physicians.

> What would have happened if—instead of these [wealthy] boys, whose families generally were able to pay for their years of study—others of less fortunate means had just finished their schooling and were beginning the exercise of their profession? What would have occurred if two or three hundred peasants had emerged, let us say by magic, from the university halls?

He goes on to predict the success of the future Cuban medical system—and to note how the development of free medical schools would make it possible for rural Cubans, and poor people around the world, to get excellent care from physicians who actually understood and respected their circumstances.

---

19   Ernesto Che Guevara and Cintio Vitie, *The Motorcycle Diaries: A Journey Around South America* (Ocean Press, 2003).

What would have happened, simply, is that the peasants would have run, immediately and with unreserved enthusiasm, to help their brothers. They would have requested the most difficult and responsible jobs in order to demonstrate that the years of study they had received had not been given in vain. What would have happened is what will happen in six or seven years, when the new students, children of workers and peasants, receive professional degrees of all kinds.

The extraordinary thing is that this poetic doctor's vision came to life. Within ten years of Guevara's speech, there were fifty-three rural hospitals in Cuba instead of one.[20] Over the next fifty years, while operating on a shoestring budget and under a strict US embargo, Cuba opened twenty-one free medical schools, four free dental schools, and four free nursing schools across the country.[21] It's no wonder that every clinic I went to had at least one wall with an iconic Warholian poster of Che Guevara in his revolutionary beret.

Society as Medicine
Che Guevara's vision, the Cuban health-care system, and the medical diplomacy program that grew from it (see below) all reflect the influence of "Social Medicine"—a concept defined by a nineteenth-century European physician named Rudolph Virchow. Virchow noted that certain epidemics were "artificial epidemics," because they arose primarily from social inequalities, and would not take such a toll if those inequalities were addressed—and that medicine should therefore focus on something broader than the pathogen alone. [22]

---

20 C. William Keck and Gail A. Reed, "The Curious Case of Cuba," *American Journal of Public Health* 102, no. 8 (2012).

21 "Health Statistics Yearbook 2005," MINSAP Cuban Ministry of Health, accessed September 27, 2012, http://www.medicc.org/publications/cuba_health_reports/cuba-health-data.php.MINSAP.

22 George Rosen, *From Medical Police to Social Medicine: Essays on the History of Health Care* (New York: Science History Publications, 1974).

In Cuba, health care became a constitutional right, as well as an international obligation. Cuban law includes the following principles in the 1976 Constitution and the 1983 Public Health Law:

- Health care is a right, available to all equally and free of charge.
- Health care is the responsibility of the state.
- Preventive and curative services are integrated.
- The public participates in the health system's development and functioning.
- Health-care activities are integrated with economic and social development.
- Global health cooperation is a fundamental obligation of the health system and its professionals.[23]

By 2012, the number of doctors in Cuba had climbed from the 3,400 doctors who had stayed after the revolution to 78,000—with 15,000 stationed overseas in Cuba's medical diplomacy program.[24] Tens of thousands of Cubans are also enrolled in free programs in nursing, dentistry, and other health professions.

This "medical economy" (and political philosophy) has created a generation of doctors and other health professionals who work for "laborer's wages."

The International Free Medical School

Cuba opened an international free medical school, known as ELAM (an acronym for Escuela Latinoamericana de Medicina, or Latin American Medical School), in 1999. It started as a simple scholarship program for 500 medical students per year from Caribbean countries that had been devastated by Hurricanes Mitch

23 C. William Keck and Gail A. Reed, "The Curious Case of Cuba," *American Journal of Public Health* 102, no. 8 (2012).
24 Elizabeth Newhouse, "Disaster Medicine: US Doctors Examine Cuba's Approach," Center for International Policy, July 9, 2012.

and George. It quickly became a full-fledged medical school in its own right that is now fully accredited and recognized by the World Health Organization and the California Board of Medicine (the strictest in the US).

The program offers six years of medical school (preceded by a 20-month intensive training in Spanish for those who need it), free room and board (though the rooms are crowded and the food is not fancy), school supplies, books, and a small monthly stipend. These scholarships are offered with the stipulation that the students receiving them will return to practice medicine in the poor and underserved areas they come from. When I was there, the doors had just barely opened, but by 2015, close to 25,000 students from eighty-four countries had graduated—all on full scholarships— including many students from underserved areas in the United States.[25] The idea is spreading. Venezuela has opened a sister school with more than 20,000 students.

The Health Studies Laboratory
It's not surprising to me that Cuba is considered by some to be the most feminist country in Latin America—women make up 43 percent of their parliament—and I wonder if this has influenced the culture of medicine.[26,27] Everywhere I went I met intelligent, confident women who were working in high ranks in medicine and public health. Sonia Baez was one of them. I was very lucky that a colleague gave me her name, literally the night before I left, when I didn't have a single contact lined up. Extremely smart, warm, and overworked, Baez—a vegetarian and meditator—is involved in virtually every sector of Cuba's health-care system. She travels internationally to find new (non-Soviet) suppliers of raw materials for Cuba's pharmaceutical industry—she recently sent me an email

25 Historia de la ELAM, http://instituciones.sld.cu/elam/historia-de-la-elam/.
26 Luisita Lopez Torregrosa, "Cuba May Be the Most Feminist Country in Latin America," *New York Times* IHT Rendezvous Blog, May 1, 2012.
27 Fidel Castro called for women's rights as a "Revolution within a revolution."

with a photo of herself riding a yak in Tibet. At the time of my visit, she also oversaw innovative organic farms where medicinal herbs were grown, and practiced acupressure and healing touch at a community-health research project called the Laboratorio de Estudios de Salud (Health Studies Laboratory).

The Laboratorio opened in 1993 and began offering free acupuncture to the community right away. "At first people were very suspicious of acupuncture," explained Lazaro Hernandez, the earnest and soft-spoken acupuncturist I met with, "but eventually we had lines forming outside as people waited for a treatment. Hospitals refer many patients here, and people also come by themselves for all kinds of problems."

When I dropped in to see the Laboratorio, they were preparing to launch a new preventive health project. An acupressure training was in session as we walked through the building, and Hernandez showed me where they would be teaching tai chi and breathing exercises to the community, as well as nutrition and health-food cooking classes. The thirty-two people who worked at the Laboratorio came from a variety of professions—family doctors, surgeons, psychologists, even an architect and a historian—many of them holding full-time jobs elsewhere. A strong culture of volunteerism, called "lending of services," makes this sort of project possible.

"We are trying to involve the whole community in this project," Hernandez said. "We are making contacts with the local school, vegetable markets . . . Ultimately we'd even like to open a health-food restaurant here, and use it as a teaching resource."

A Prison Turns into an Alternative Medicine Polyclinic

The next day I took a painfully slow old train (with floppy seat backs that had lost their ability to stand up) to visit a clinic that Sonia Baez had told me I *must* see, in Matanzas, a city about two hours outside of Havana.

Matanzas, Cuba's oldest city, has an eerie feel to it. The name Matanzas, which means "of the killing," was first penned on a map in 1526, in reference to an incident in which the indigenous nationals overturned canoes of thirty invading Spaniards. Because of their heavy metal armor, the Spaniards drowned easily. But that didn't stop Spain. In the 1800s, the vast majority of the city's population were African slaves imported by Spaniards to work on the sugar plantations.[28]

The clinic there had a few ghosts of its own. It was in a large building that had served as a jail during the pre-revolution Batista regime. "Prisoners were beaten and tortured here under Batista, and now . . ." said Gladys Rodriguez, who was showing me around, as she swept her hand down a long brown-and-yellow hallway filled with benches and doorways. Each doorway had a sign sticking out: "Massage," "Acupuncture," "Herbal Medicine," "Magnet Therapy," "Psychotherapy," "Homeopathy"—the list of available treatments went on and on. It seemed indulgent, until I remembered that Cuban patients pay the same amount for an acupuncture treatment or a massage as they do for open heart surgery: absolutely nothing.

The doctor who founded the polyclinic, Juventino Acosta Meir, was presenting a paper at an international conference in Africa the week I visited, so I didn't get to meet him. The doctors I did meet kept asking me, "Have you met Juventino?" with a sparkle in their eyes. "He's quite something," they said, "you'll have to come back." He had been the chief of urology at the large provincial hospital, but left that position to start the polyclinic in 1994. The polyclinic was one of the first to use an integrative approach to treatment, combining standard and alternative modalities. His colleagues back at the hospital were skeptical, but within the first year the new integrative clinic had already served 23,000 patients, getting excellent results on a relatively small budget, so they were allowed to continue. By the time I visited they were seeing more than 50,000 people per year.

During much of the day, the Matanzas clinic doubles as a senior center. The hallways are filled with elders keeping each other company as they wait for massage, acupressure, counseling, and

28 Laird W. Bergad, *Cuban Rural Society in the Nineteenth Century: The Social and Economic History of Monoculture in Matanzas* (Princeton, NJ: Princeton University Press, 1990).

general health care. The clinic arranges rides in from the countryside for them on Red Cross buses in the morning, and back to their
neighborhoods and outlying small towns later in the afternoon,
saving fuel and building connections.

The same clinic runs children's educational programs every day
after school. Small groups of ten-, eleven-, and twelve-year-olds
come one afternoon a week (100 children in all) to study herbal
medicine, nutrition, sex education, tai chi, painting, poetry, and
music. A group of twelve children with Down's syndrome also
comes to the clinic three days a week for therapy and classes.

This "stacking of functions" in one large building has secondary
benefits: it creates opportunities for conversation and connections
to develop between people who might otherwise be isolated by age,
illness, or disability. And less time and resources are spent on maintenance, cleaning, and temperature control than if each program
were happening in its own building.

Most of the fifty-seven physicians who work in the polyclinic have
an additional degree in natural and traditional medicine. One of
them, an anesthesiologist named Dr. Lazara Blanco, had originally
trained with doctors from China in 1977. She said that because of
supply-chain issues with anesthetic drugs, she had routinely used
acupuncture in place of anesthesia for thyroid, mastectomy, and
uterine fibroid surgeries, but she never thought they would end up
relying on it so much for standard care.

Since 1994, training in acupuncture has been integrated into the
medical school curriculum in Cuba. For example, acupuncture point
location is taught within the basic anatomy curriculum, and pattern-
based Chinese medical physiology is taught along with standard
Western physiology. Every medical student also does a clinical rota-
tion in natural and traditional medicine, and can go on to specialize
in it with four additional years of training past the MD degree.[29]

---

29 Harriet Beinfield, "Dreaming with Two Feet on the Ground: Acupuncture in Cuba,"
    Clinical Acupuncture and Oriental Medicine, June 2, 2001.

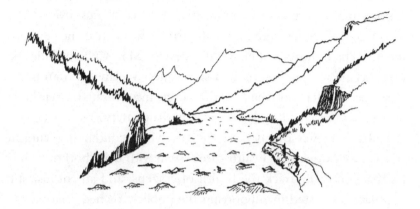

Developing Medications for
Themselves and the World

Back in Havana, I met with a husband-and-wife doctor team who worked at a large hospital. Over lunch, they rattled off numerous pharmaceutical research projects that they were involved in. Typical of the country's triaging of resources, the Cubans were making their own pharmaceuticals even while they were running short on glass bottles to dispense them in.

Rather than relying on foreign manufacturers for drugs, dozens of research and production facilities in Cuba now produce 83 percent of the medications used in their own country. Cuba has found a niche by creating new drugs and vaccines that target diseases of poor and developing nations—the kind of drug research and development that private pharmaceutical corporations avoid because it is unprofitable. Because Cuba's drug development programs are in the public sector, they can afford to make different choices. Cuba sells its pharmaceuticals on an international sliding scale—providing them at a profit to countries that can afford to pay for them, and to poorer countries at little or no charge.[30]

---

30 Gerry Bill, "Priorities: Cuba Continues to Develop Health and Education for the People," *Pacific Free Press*, September 6, 2011.

Although we hear little about it in the United States, Cuba exports pharmaceuticals to more than fifty countries around the world and is known internationally for its work in drug development.[31] The hundreds of new drugs developed in Cuba include the first vaccine for Meningitis B, a skin-cancer vaccine, and an influenza vaccine that, for the first time ever, incorporated a synthetic antigen (considered a major advance in drug safety).[32,33]

Cuba has two distinct advantages when conducting clinical trials: a well-organized health-care system with neighborhood clinics that can easily track the health of citizens, and an enthusiastic populace interested in supporting the publicly owned pharmaceutical sector—knowing that the profits will circulate back into their own health-care system.

Cuban research is generally not published in US medical journals, nor have Cuban pharmaceuticals been easily available here, partly because of the embargo. (One notable exception to this is a US drug company that was able to work around the embargo by paying in supplies, rather than cash, for partial rights to a skin-cancer vaccine that Cuba developed.)[34]

A National Experiment in Homeopathic Vaccines

Cuba successfully produced a short-acting human vaccine for a water-borne illness called leptospirosis—an illness that can become epidemic during floods, and is increasing in incidence as the climate shifts. It is caused by a spirochete (like syphilis and Lyme disease) that is transmitted through animal urine as floodwater spreads it around the landscape. It starts with flu-like symptoms, but if

31 John M. Kirk and H. Michael Erisman, *Cuban Medical Internationalism: Origins, Evolution, and Goals* (New York: Palgrave Macmillan, 2009).
32 Halla Thorsteinsdottir, et al., "Cuba—Innovation Through Synergy," *Nature Biotechnology* 22 (2004).
33 V. Verez-Bencomo, et al., "A Synthetic Conjugate Polysaccharide Vaccine Against Haemophilus Influenzae Type B," *Science* 5 (2004):305–522.
34 Penni Crabtree, "Carlsbad Biotech in Cancer Deal with Cuba," *Union-Tribune*, July 15, 2004.

left untreated it can lead to meningitis, respiratory problems, and kidney failure. Cuba, being an island in the Southern Hemisphere, deals with outbreaks of leptospirosis regularly. After Cuba was hit hard by three hurricanes in a row in 2007, the Cuban Ministry of Public Health only had enough vaccine left to treat 15,000 people. So they decided to try something new: they conducted an enormous experimental campaign using homeopathic medicine.

The homeopathic research drug was given to a total of 2.3 million people in the provinces that tend to be most affected, making this the largest homeopathic research study ever. Out of every 100,000 people treated, only four got leptospirosis, compared with the typical thirty-eight per week during that time of year.[35] Among the 8.8 million people in the other provinces who did not receive homeopathic treatment, the incidence of leptospirosis was as high as was predicted based on rainfall. The effect appeared to be sustained: there was an 84 percent reduction in infection in the homeopathically treated region in the following year (2008), while in the same period, incidence in the untreated region increased by 22 percent.[36, 37] Their willingness to try out-of-the-box approaches successfully reduced the spread of leptospirosis—and for a fraction of what vaccines normally cost them each year.

Medical Diplomacy

Cuba uses the overflow from its free medical schools to provide care internationally, by offering "medical diplomacy" (free medical

---

35 Lionel R. Milgrom, Maria R. Ringo, and Karen M. Wehrstein, "Emerging Economies' Need for Cheap, Efficient Health Care Makes Western Anti-Homeopathy Rhetoric Irrelevant: Observations from the Canadian Homeopathy Conference, October 2011," *Journal of Alternative and Complementary Medicine* 18, no 7 (2012):1–4.

36 Gustavo Bracho, et al., "Large-Scale Application of Highly-Diluted Bacteria for Leptospirosis Epidemic Control," *Homeopathy* 99 (2010):156–66.

37 "Homeopathy Associated with Dramatic Reduction in Leptospirosis Infection in Cuban Population," *Medical News Today*, August 9, 2010, http://www.medicalnewstoday.com/articles/197128.php.

care and medications) to countries in need. At last count, Cuba had 35,000 medical workers providing care in more than 70 countries to some 70 million patients.[38] Thousands of children suffering from radiation poisoning in Chernobyl were flown in and treated for free each year in Cuba.

Cuba, a tiny nation of 11 million, has the largest medical emergency response corps on standby in the world.[39] They sent 2,500 medical professionals to Pakistan after the massive earthquake in 2005. They stayed for six months, worked in 44 locations, cared for more than a million people, and performed 12,400 operations. When they left, they donated all the equipment from the thirty-two field hospitals they had set up, and offered medical school scholarships to 1,000 Pakistani youths with the understanding that, once they graduated, they would return to Pakistan to treat their own people.[40]

Julie Feinsilver, author of *Healing the Masses: Cuban Health Politics at Home and Abroad*, notes that Cuban doctors often work in remote areas providing services that the host population has never seen. In fifteen months in Iraq from 1984 to 1985, Cuban doctors attended more than a million patients on an outpatient basis, performed 1,743 surgeries, and assisted 3,700 births. A team of 182 medical workers, mostly women, stayed in Iraq to continue to provide aid in Iraqi hospitals during the Persian Gulf War when all other international medical aid teams had left. Cubans also helped to develop the Children's Orthopedic Hospital in Bagdad, where sixty-seven Cubans were on staff in 1988. During eight years of the Iran–Iraq war, the staff there attended more than 25,000 children and performed 10,000 pediatric surgeries.[41]

In another case, in 1999, Cuba sent 234 medical professionals and thirty-five literacy teachers to work in East Timor, knowing

38   John M. Kirk and H. Michael Erisman, *Cuban Medical Internationalism: Origins, Evolution, and Goals* (New York: Palgrave MacMillan, 2009).
39   Ibid., 178.
40   Ibid., 176.
41   Julie Margot Feinsilver, *Healing the Masses: Cuban Health Politics at Home and Abroad* (Berkeley: University of California Press, 1993).

that after years of violence, there were only thirty-five physicians left there. Within six years infant mortality rates were reduced by 50 percent. As the health of the country stabilized, the Cubans then set about training new doctors for East Timor—689 of them attended the free medical school in Cuba, and 148 more were trained in East Timor itself—to replenish the country's supply of physicians.[42]

Sometimes Cuba's aid is not accepted. In 2005, Cuban doctors waited for days at the airport in Havana, with their backpacks, ready to help out during the aftermath of Hurricane Katrina in New Orleans, to see if the US would allow them entry. Castro offered Louisiana 1,586 Cuban doctors, as well as portable field hospitals and many tons of medical supplies,[43] saying that in these circumstances, no matter how rich the country, "it was clear to us that what was needed were young, well-trained and experienced professionals who had done medical work in anomalous circum-stances."[44] Given their experience in underserved areas and natural disasters, and the proximity of Cuba to New Orleans (less than 700 miles—a 90-minute flight), it should have been a no-brainer. President Bush refused them, despite Bush's assurances that accep-tance of international aid offers would be kept free of politics.

When necessary, Cuban doctors will work at many levels of a country's health-care system in order to deal with a crisis. The Gambian president invited a team of Cuban specialists to provide advice on the epidemic of malaria in Gambia, which was the number one killer in the country. In addition to working directly with patients, the Cuban doctors worked as advisors in the Ministry of Public Health and in programs to combat malaria, as well as

42 John M. Kirk and H. Michael Erisman, *Cuban Medical Internationalism: Origins, Evolution, and Goals* (New York: Palgrave MacMillan, 2009).
43 Mary Murray, "Katrina Aid from Cuba? No Thanks, Says US," NBCNews.com, September 14, 2005.
44 Remarks by Dr. Fidel Castro Ruz, President of the Republic of Cuba, meeting with the medical doctors assembled to offer assistance to the American people in areas affected by Hurricane Katrina, Havana Convention Center, September 4, 2005, http://www.cuba.cu/gobierno/discursos/2005/ing/f040905i.html.

tuberculosis and HIV/AIDS. They launched several key initiatives, including the creation of a national reference library for clinical and laboratory research, the use of a new biolarvicide (developed in Cuba), and in-depth training for Gambian health professionals, including a semester of medical entomology for nursing, public health, and medical students. Within two years, cases of malaria in Gambia went down from 600,000 to 200,000.[45]

A Medical Draft?

Why do Cuban doctors do this work? In an interview, Cuba's Deputy Minister Jimenez, discussing whether medical internationalism was carried out solely to garner international support, turned the tables on the questioner. "Even taking the most cynical view, namely that Cuba is sending doctors abroad to poor countries in order to win votes at the UN, why doesn't the industrialized world do something similar? Surely the most important thing is to save lives. That is precisely what our policy is doing."[46]

Critics have said that Cuban doctors are "forced" to do this work. It is true that the working-class salaries of Cuban doctors would not lure many people from overseas to join them. Yet from my conversations in Cuba, as well as from stories of colleagues who have worked alongside Cuban doctors overseas and during disaster relief operations, I don't think this is an accurate description of how most Cuban doctors see the situation. I think they view it more like the way most people in the United States view military service: some volunteer for military service while others are drafted, but overall the country's goal is to have a group of strong, willing young adults available to "help out" overseas, in hopes of creating a safer and more egalitarian world.

---

45 John M. Kirk and H. Michael Erisman, *Cuban Medical Internationalism: Origins, Evolution, and Goals* (New York: Palgrave MacMillan, 2009).

46 John M. Kirk and H. Michael Erisman, *Cuban Medical Internationalism: Origins, Evolution, and Goals* (New York: Palgrave MacMillan, 2009), 179.

Hurricane Preparedness in Cuba

One clear benefit this work overseas has given Cuban health professionals is that they now have vast experience in preparing for and responding to natural disasters. "Cuba is one of the best prepared, if not *the* best prepared [country] for natural disasters," UN Undersecretary-General for Humanitarian Affairs and Emergency Relief Coordinator Jan Egeland told Reuters. "The same hurricane which would take zero lives in Cuba would kill massively in Haiti."[47] The Center for International Policy notes that a person is fifteen times more likely to be killed by a hurricane in the United States than in Cuba.[48] Meteorological hurricane forecasting is a specialty of Cuba's, and it's one of the few areas where the US and Cuba have long agreed to share resources, since hurricanes generally hit Cuba just before they reach the United States. Ever since Hurricane Katrina's devastating effects on New Orleans, US officials have been visiting Cuba to learn better hurricane preparedness strategies from them.[49]

Disaster-response training in Cuba starts in childhood as part of the school curriculum and continues with adult education at the community level. Disaster medicine is also a substantial part of standard training for all health-care professionals.[50] More than 95 percent of the population has been trained in a four-step framework: information, alert, alarm, and recovery. Two-day community-level simulations happen each May, before the storms build up. People discuss their roles in various possible scenarios and then practice evacuations, including skills like cutting tree branches. As a result, virtually all Cubans understand weather warnings and know their

47 Lilja Otto, "Cuba's Hurricane Resilience: Solidarity and Readiness," *Yes! Magazine*, May 10, 2006.
48 Elizabeth Newhouse, "Disaster Medicine: US Doctors Examine Cuba's Approach," Center for International Policy, July 9, 2012.
49 Jean Friedman-Rudovsky, "Hurricane Tips from Cuba," *New York Times*, July 29, 2013.
50 Elizabeth Newhouse, "Disaster Medicine: US Doctors Examine Cuba's Approach," Center for International Policy, July 9, 2012.

expected roles during every stage of a storm. Every neighborhood knows who will stay where during a storm, and who is in charge of helping the neighbors with disabilities or families with multiple children.[51]

Cuba's Environmental Revolution

"We are not waiting for fuel to fall from the sky, because we have discovered, fortunately, something much more important— energy conservation, which is like finding a great oil deposit."

—**Fidel Castro, in his May 2006 address to the Cuban Electric Utility company (UNE)**

In 1959, the Cuban landscape was scarred by centuries of environmental degradation rooted in colonialism. Plantation owners had cut down forests to plant coffee, sugar, and tobacco and reap huge profits, with a resulting loss of biodiversity, local food security, and topsoil. The first agrarian reforms after the revolution in Cuba reflected an environmental consciousness on the part of the new Cuban government. The reforms protected topsoil, set aside tracts of conservation land, and conserved swamps and wetlands in hopes of saving endangered species there. Some of these reforms made a huge difference in Cuba's development: the coastline, in particular, being publicly owned, is far better protected from development than it is on most island nations. The coastal wetlands are an enormously beneficial carbon sink, and also serve as a buffer against hurricane damage.

Those reforms, however, weren't enough to resuscitate Cuba's farmland. For a few decades, Cuba tried to emulate Soviet industrial development, with massive nationalized farms using large machin-

---

51 Lilja Otto, "Cuba's Hurricane Resilience—Solidarity and Readiness," *Yes! Magazine*, May 10, 2006.

ery and large amounts of pesticides and fertilizers. They continued to grow sugarcane, exporting it to the USSR.

When the USSR collapsed, however, the Soviet industrial agricultural approach quickly gave way to organic farming, with more sustainable methods—by necessity if not by choice. This translated to far less machinery, natural pest and weed control, use of compost and manure rather than chemical fertilizers, and a switch to smaller, more localized farming cooperatives. Cuban farmers soon saw the benefits—more satisfying human-scaled work, more and better food in each local region, and fewer pollutants in the water and soil.[52]

Around the time of my visit, a second revolution was brewing in Cuba. Castro had attended the world summit in Rio de Janeiro in 1996, and Cuba was among the first countries to embrace the biodiversity measures proposed there. The government identified seventeen endangered ecosystems on the island and began carrying out measures to protect them. Castro delivered a speech calling for less consumerism and a more equal distribution of the world's resources in order to preserve the world's natural environment.[53]

A few years later, Castro decreed an "Energy Revolution" to decrease Cuba's dependence on fossil fuels. They imported a million bicycles and built five bicycle factories. They replaced nearly every light bulb in the country and updated millions of household appliances. They built wind farms and solar farms. Animal waste was recycled to create biogas, and sugarcane waste became biomass fuel. They built microhydro generators to harness the natural energy of streams and rivers, installed thousands of emergency backup systems, and separated out the massive national grid into smaller local grids that would not impact each other during power outages.[54]

52 John Bachtell, "Cuba Constructs Environmentally Sustainable Socialism," *People's World,* September 5, 2009.
53 Ibid.
54 "La Revolucion Energetica: Cuba's Energy Revolution," renewableenergyworld. com, April 9, 2009.

Although progress was sometimes bumpy, and some citizens complained about the measures, Cuba was able to reduce its energy consumption dramatically, using only 34 percent of the kerosene (for cooking), 40 percent of the LPG (liquefied petroleum gas), and 80 percent of the gasoline it had consumed before the implementation of the energy revolution a mere two years earlier.

By 2008, each Cuban citizen was responsible for only 2.1 tons of CO_2e in the atmosphere each year (compared to 20.1 tons per capita in the US). Cuba is the only country in the world that has a sustainable ecological footprint while still meeting the United Nations' criteria for a high Human Development Index (life expectancy, literacy, education, and per capita GDP).[55,56]

Rather than having less energy available to the public after these conservation measures, the country actually has far more energy, and more reliable energy. All the rural schools, public buildings, and clinics that needed electricity were updated with solar power systems, and most areas of the country that didn't have electricity now do. Between 2004 and 2007, blackouts lasting an hour or more were reduced from 400 a year to zero.[57]

Although I initially traveled to Cuba mostly out of curiosity, the depth of what I saw there has filtered down over time, and its relevance to our current challenges has become clearer to me. I saw people working in innovative groups (despite the fact that they had little money or supplies) to build up a varied and vibrant health-care system that not only could take care of its own people, but had enough resources to spare to send doctors around the world. Cuba has created and maintained a high-quality health-care system and a high standard of health for its citizens, revamped its agricul-

---

55 WWF International, Living Planet Report 2006, http://d2ouvy59p0dg6k.cloud front.net/downloads/living_planet_report.pdf.
56 Chuluun Togtoch and Owen Gaffney, 2010 Human Sustainable Development Index, Our World, United Nations University, http://ourworld.unu.edu/en/the-2010-human-sustainable-development-index.
57 "La Revolucion Energetica: Cuba's Energy Revolution," renewableenergyworld .com, April 9, 2009.

tural system, and extended generosity out to the world on a budget that is just a fraction of our own, with a truly sustainable carbon footprint. They have done this while petroleum-based resources are scarce, economics are shaky, and hurricanes are picking up speed—conditions much like those we are starting to encounter around the world.

Whatever you might think about Cuban politics, Cuba is a useful example of what the transition to a different way of living could be like. Whether by choice or by necessity, Cuba's response to a nation-wide crisis shows just how quickly and effectively large-scale adaptation can happen, in a nation that has put health care, environment, and education at the top of its priorities.

Perhaps the biggest lesson I learned from Cuba is that a national (or international) health-care system does not need to be fueled by petroleum, profits, cutting-edge technology, or elitism in order to be effective; rather, it can rely on everyday working-class people, trusting in their innate compassion, generosity, creativity, and intelligence.

Flying Home

As I flew back from Cuba, I picked up a *Glamour* magazine tucked into the seatback in front of me. Flipping through it, I came across a full-page ad of a gorgeous model wearing expensive leather boots. Staring at the picture, I felt a sensation rising up in me: *"I want those. If I had them I would be happy."*

And then I burst into tears. Not because of the boots, but because I realized that within half an hour of being back in the world of consumerism, *it* was back. A kind of covetous desire I hadn't felt the entire time I had been in Cuba. I had never really noticed it before, but now it was right in my face.

Of course Cubans are not immune to material desires—far from it. But for a week I had been in a country where there was no advertising, and not much of anything to buy other than the essentials: food, medicine, a few books, handmade art, and simple clothing. It was the first time I had been on a trip where shopping was not an option. In its place there was live music, dancing, and deep conversation. There were people offering rides to strangers, rebuilding a local food system, and using their ingenuity in fixing everything from old cars to X-ray machines.

Seeing that flash of longing for luxurious boots against a backdrop of the deep human satisfaction I had felt in Cuba was the contrast I needed. It allowed me to see something that operates all the time when I'm living in the United States: the thing that constantly drives me to want new things to eat, new clothes to wear, new technology to use. It's especially striking because I live a virtually media-free life in Vermont—I don't watch TV, there are no billboards, and I rarely read glitzy magazines. But in a growth economy, the drive toward spending more and having more is built right in to our consciousness by the time we learn how toddle toward our first toys. The ads I saw as a young person are still doing their work.

Merchandising nowadays is built into the products themselves, carefully crafted by market researchers and psychologists who are paid to figure out what appeals to our instinctual desires. Even in a rural town in Vermont, the clothes I see my neighbors wearing and the cars I see them driving all say to me "if you had this, you would be happier."

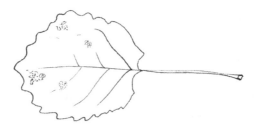

CHAPTER NINE

The Commons of Care

"There is nobility in the duty to care for creation through little daily actions . . . We must not think that these efforts are not going to change the world. They benefit society, often unbeknown to us, for they call forth a goodness which, albeit unseen, inevitably tends to spread."

—**Pope Francis,** *Laudato Si*

D ifferent societies have different ways of recognizing the basic reality that, actually, everything belongs to everyone.

In hunting and herding cultures like those of the Inuit or Mongolians, land, grass, trees, ice, and water are (or were) all part of the "commons"—shared among the humans and animals who roam through the area. Certain groups may control certain territories, but within those groups, resources are generally shared. When the linguist Daniel Everett visited the Piraha, a Brazilian hunting culture, he was surprised to see that after a large kill, the hunters would share the animal with everyone in the village without storing any for later.

"Why don't you store the meat?" Everett asked.

"I store meat in the belly of my brother," the hunter answered.[1]

In many towns in Mexico, the staple crops of corn and beans are raised in commonly owned fields that are harvested for the community. If it's a fruitful year, then everyone has a lot to eat. If it's a slim year, no one does—but at least everyone has a little. In certain

1   Charles Eisenstein, Lecture, Goddard College, February 2012.

wilderness areas in the Ukraine, anyone can build a cabin to live in. Groups of people all over the world share nonmaterial things as well: languages, jokes, traditions, fairy tales, and more recently, the Internet, open-source software, and Wikipedia.

Gradually, over the course of history, there has been an increasing privatization of commonly held resources. Rich growing areas, grazing areas, and forests have been carved up, with ownership given to individuals—usually those who were in favor with the powers that be, rather than the people who had been using them communally for generations.

This "enclosure of the commons" has implications that we are only beginning to understand. From the prairies of America to the steppes of Russia, guns and fences have stopped the migration of massive herds of wild grazing animals across the continents, as well as the predators that kept those herds from overgrazing in any one area. Once predator and prey were gone, we lost nearly everything that depended on their presence and movement: grasslands, topsoil, soil organisms, soil fertility, carbon and water cycling, and biological diversity. All of these losses affect our health.

The growth economy puts increasing pressure on natural resources as people try to find new things to sell. Landowners, communities, and even nations are selling mining, gas, and oil rights on their land. Now, even water rights are up for sale. On a global scale, as corporations use their financial influence to lobby for looser environmental regulations, we are quickly losing the most basic "commons" that we used to be able to depend on: a stable climate, sparkling clear underground aquifers, oceans full of fish, even the shapes of mountains.

In the desperation of a faltering economy, people are patenting everything—from ancient yoga poses to traditional seed varieties, to genetic codes of beneficial bacteria—with lawsuits and fines levied on those who use them without paying for permission.

Yet there have always been some people keeping an eye on the commons, and making sure that certain parts of life do not get privatized, understanding that everyone benefits when certain resources are shared. In Massachusetts, where I grew up, reservoirs of drinking water are shared by all who live near them, and we knew as children that we were expected not to swim in them, in order to keep the water as clean as possible. Here in Thetford, we have a town forest as a backup reservoir of firewood.

Many things are still part of the commons, even in our capitalist economy—with shared costs, governance, and upkeep, as well as widespread benefit. In neighborhoods we share community gardens, playgrounds, athletic fields, public beaches, and houses of worship. In most communities our schools, fire departments, buses, subways, libraries, parks, sewers, roads, reservoirs, sidewalks, police departments, postal service, trash collection, and more are all part of the "public works" or "common good." Everyone benefits from having roads without potholes, and working sewers, so everyone who can afford to pays for them, one way or another.

In all these cases of the commons, people may disagree about the best use of the shared resource, but it's generally accepted that no one should be making a profit off the venture.

What we share in the United States seems normal to us, and we look down on cultures that don't have good public works. It seems strange, then, that so many Americans are threatened by the idea of making health care part of the public works or "commons." They struggle with the idea of nationalized or single-payer health care, thinking that it would mean that the US was Socialist, or worse, Communist.

Should Health Care Be Part of the Commons?

In the vast majority of "developed" countries (yes, capitalist ones too), health care is part of the commons—available to everyone, with the costs shared by all members of society. People who live in Europe, Asia, Canada, and other places where medical care is part

of the public works look at our health-care system with its varying rules, price structures, deductibles, paperwork, waiting periods,
fees, and ways of excluding people who are actually sick, and think
it is bizarre.

I love the scene in Michael Moore's movie *Sicko* in which Moore
is in an English hospital, trying to find the billing department. He
goes from door to door, hallway to hallway, asking. Everyone insists
there is no billing department, because there are no bills to be sent
out to patients or insurance companies. Doctors and nurses are
simply paid a salary and do their job. Finally, he finds a man standing in a little bank-teller type room with a sign that says "cashier,"
and Moore says, "Aha!" The man does deal in money. But it turns
out his only job is to give out cash to people without cars who can't
afford a taxi ride home from the hospital.

In countries like England that have a true national health service
(as opposed to requirements that all citizens buy private health
insurance), no one deals with billing and insurance codes in the
world of medicine: patients don't, administrative assistants don't,
and doctors don't either. Everyone involved can simply focus on
giving and receiving care. It is hard to imagine. But it is a choice we
could make in the United States.

In countries like Cuba where everyone has a primary care team
living right in the neighborhood, free of charge and accessible at
all hours, it seems just as normal to them as having a nearby fire
department, available at any hour, does to us. No one in the United
States ever suggests that we should not pitch in to pay for the fire
department, because we all understand that any of us could need
them at any time. The same is actually true of health-care providers.
If your house is burning, you need the fire department. If you are
sick, you need care.

How would you feel if your rich neighbors got firefighters to
come right away, but your "firefighter policy" had a ten-hour waiting period and a $5,000 deductible? What if people who had already
had a fire in the past were excluded by the fire department because

of "prior conditions"? What if your poor neighbors couldn't afford the fire department's exorbitant fees at all?

Of course it wouldn't be fair. But if something is part of a culture for long enough, even if it doesn't make sense, it eventually becomes "normal." In subtle and not-so-subtle ways, people learn "it has always been that way in our culture," and over time, we integrate it into our view of how reality has to be. We get other false messages like: "There just isn't enough to go around, so someone has to lose out."

The simple truth is that there is money to be made by keeping health care in the private sector, and those who are already invested in the health-care industry are spending some of their profits on making sure that things don't change.

The Loss of the Social Commons of Care

The competitive mentality of the growth economy has affected another aspect of the commons: the "social commons." Earlier I showed how the AMA created restrictive licensing and competitive education for certain types of doctors while scaring people away from the "quackery" of other types of care—thereby narrowing the medical field into a profitable monoculture. Similarly, other groups have created professional licensing—and profitable business models—that take over roles that traditionally were part of the commons, while using advertising to scare people into using those services. We gradually get trained to think it is normal to pay for many things that, in other cultures, are part of the commons, including things like people helping each other, healing each other, massaging each other, playing with children, and caring for elders.[2]

For example, as Charles Eisenstein noted, if you scare people away from touching each other without a license, there is more money to

2   Charles Eisenstein, Lecture, Goddard College, February 2012.

be made for those who are licensed, but there is a huge loss in the valuable social commons of warm, caring contact and healing touch. In theory, acknowledging a certain level of skill, experience, or training is a good thing, but when it is combined with a profit-driven competitive market it can work against community-based values of people helping and trusting each other.

The loss of the social commons is an exponential problem. If most parents have been scared out of letting children play in the woods, and have been convinced to pay for camps and after-school enrichment programs instead, then the child who stays home in the summers has no one to play with. There are no packs of roving children playing in the brook at the edge of the field and woods, and no stickball games in the street, so the bored child in the living room (whose parents can't afford camp) becomes a bother. So for the families that can't afford camps there is another product to buy: video games that simulate playing. With some children in camps, and others plugged in to video games, the grandparent at home has less to do and less to contribute, and starts to feel like they are a drain on the family. So now an institution advertises that they will take care of our elders, and suddenly it seems worth it.

The more of a sense we have that our needs, our disabilities, and our illnesses are bothersome, irritating, or a drain on our friends and family, the more we are willing to pay someone to take care of us (and the more normal we think it is to move people to nursing homes or institutions when they become "too much of a bother"). The advertisements that promote health-care institutions (as well as other service industries, such as hair dressers, therapists, dog-walking services, and day-care centers) serve as a constant reminder that it is important not to depend too heavily on friends, family, and neighbors.

In our current health-care system, help, care, and attention are things that we need to pay for, and pay a *lot* for. The costs of all of these services rise over time, especially as other options fall away (and we forget they ever existed). That's partly because, increasingly, care is seen as a one-way relationship. Counseling, medical care, nursing, therapeutic touch, education, haircuts, carpentry, and all the rest, are things that we *get* from someone, but we never give back to the *same person*. We are given subtle messages by the increasing profes- sionalization of care that there is something intrinsically wrong with sharing care back and forth—that laypeople are "unprofessional" and therefore poorly trained, unskilled, and untrustworthy.

In end-stage capitalism, everything becomes a commodity. Payment is expected everywhere—and very little happens just for the sheer joy of it.

"Fix Me": Our Addiction to Professional Health Care

We have created a nation of people who are "addicted" to health care—convinced that doctors, psychiatrists, medication, or surgery can "solve" almost any problem. In a for-profit system, there is a benefit when those who are using the care are dependent on it. Here are some of the symptoms of our addiction:

- Lack of trust and understanding that many conditions get better on their own
- Fewer coping skills for dealing with (or helping others deal with) emotional or physical discomfort
- Increased use of over-the-counter drugs that quickly address symptoms without addressing the underlying cause
- Rising costs, as there is more "need" for care
- Lack of knowledge, trust, and willingness among laypeople or family members to care for others: every- thing needs to get checked by a doctor
- Loss of home-based health-care and counseling skills due to lack of practice, so less care is available in the community

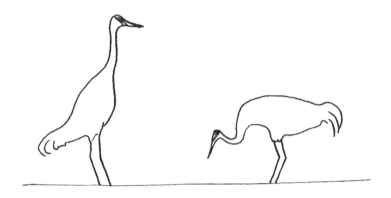

The Health-Care Underground:
Mothers and Other Unnoticed Providers

In uncertain economic times, it makes sense to be sharing resources, including the resource of care. What was once an intrinsic part of a community—people taking turns looking out for each other's emotional and physical well-being—can be revived and relearned. Building real connections with each other, including the willingness to care for each other's bodies, is an essential part of developing resiliency in our communities. Our first step in that direction may be remembering how valuable family and community-based caregivers are.

Susun Weed, in her book *Healing Wise*, notes that up to 99 percent of all health care provided worldwide is done by mothers who care for their families' health, and most of this is done in traditional "wise woman" ways. But since this is not measured by experts, or paid for, it is invisible. Preventive care in general, especially the kind that is done in people's homes—cooking healthy meals, listening, encouraging, and creating safe and supportive environments—is invisible, as well.

In *All That We Share,* author Jay Walljasper writes of caregivers as a sort of "commons" whose resources, in an extractive economy, can be used up if they are not well tended to. Everyone who helps take care of children, family members, and sick and elderly neighbors for little or no pay can be seen as part of our commons (sometimes referred to as our "social capital"). This means that within a community, there must be a conscious effort to make sure that people like parents—who are caring for others on an ongoing basis—are well taken care of themselves, that they are not getting "used up" for lack of support. They need meals offered, dishes washed, rides offered, listening ears, hugs, appreciation, and they may need financial support, as well. Those of us who aren't full-time caregivers can rotate our own time and energy through their lives to take up some of the work, and make sure they are well cared for. Once we see them as a communal resource that benefits all of us, we will all pitch in to ensure that they thrive.

In a town where people tend to take good care of their caretakers, the effects are palpable. Parents and day-care providers are less stressed, so children entering elementary school have stronger social skills, playing well together, rarely bullying each other, and knowing how to offer each other support. This, in turn, puts less stress on families, who then have more caretaking resources to put toward the elders in town—offering free rides, help with chores, etc. The elders, feeling valued and well taken care of, have more energy to help out with the younger generation, and become part of the "commons of care."

This is like a permaculture model of care, with the outputs of one system becoming the inputs of another—a nice cycle from generation to generation.

Irrational Needs versus Rational Needs

There is an underlying assumption in a growth economy that whatever people pay for is what people want, and that whatever people want is what is best for them. Unfortunately, that is not always true.

People's wants in modern society are too often based on desires, addictions, and fears that are not always rational—many of which have been created in us by someone trying to make a profit. Our world is now made up of goods and services that are all for sale, and we have been distanced from rich interconnected relationships of helping and relying on each other. In the process, many of our real needs have fallen by the wayside.

What we actually need is close, loving connection up to the moment of our death, not endless extension of the pumping of our lungs and hearts in a room full of beeping machines. What we actually need are partners who accept the changes in our bodies and our sexuality as we grow older, not drugs that produce erections or prevent women from showing signs of menopause. What we actually need is help for families, places for wild play, and schools that support children's unique needs and learning styles, not drugs to get our children to sit still when they are anxious or bored. What we actually need is help with our addictions to sugar, alcohol, and tobacco, not more drugs and procedures to treat diabetes, lung cancer, and heart disease. But these very real and rational needs do not make a profit.

So, we have choices. We can ignore the whole thing. We can swim hard against the current and try, as individuals, to take care of each other's real needs, while still struggling to care for ourselves within a system that doesn't give us time to rest and think. Or we can work to change the system itself.

Going AWOL from the Medical-Industrial Complex

Most of our health-care system now can be considered a "medical-industrial complex." Whether you work within it, or get health care from it—even if you are the owner of a large pharmaceutical corporation—there is a sense these days of being a small cog in some huge machine that keeps you turning out whatever you turn out: doctors scheduling appointments for patients that are too short to be helpful, drug companies producing medicines that mask symptoms instead of treating the causes of illness, patients going to work when they're sick just to get their required hours in. There is a sense that your decisions are not your own; that everything else in the system is turning things in a certain predictable way, and that therefore, in order to survive, you must also participate. There is a sense of something larger operating; a sense that even if you want things to change, everything else is working against it. Yet at the same time, the huge machine is getting rusty and expensive to repair.

We can step outside the machine at any time and walk away from the whole dark and dingy factory. We do this by remembering the true roots of our health and healing: strong local communities, both human and nonhuman. There are risks, to be sure, in leaving the medical-industrial medical complex, but there are also huge benefits. As we move away from the predictable rusty grinding wheels of this technological behemoth, we step out into a bright world full of unpredictability and unknowns, as well as freshness, vitality, and infinite possibility.

Parish Nursing: A Model of Embedded Care

Just across the river from me, in Lyme, New Hampshire, Ellen Thompson is practicing an old form of medicine, where profits are not in the picture. The Lyme Congregational Church hired her to be the "parish nurse" who keeps an eye out for those who need help, not just among parishioners, but for the whole town. Like many rural New England communities, Lyme is full of fiercely independent white protestants who, while generous themselves, have a hard time asking for help, especially during long, cold winters. New Hampshire's motto "Live Free or Die" takes on a different tone for elders, who joke that what it really means is "Live, *Freeze,* and Die."

The church raises money from the community and pays Ellen about $20,000 a year. In a town of about 2,000 residents, that amounts to less than one dollar per month per person. Ellen ends up working about fifteen hours a week, at a variety of hours, though she is basically on call, as needed, to everyone in town. This works out just right for her. At age sixty-two, she was ready to retire after forty years of working long hours at a large hospital, and yet she still wanted to be of service, and she wanted to do it closer to home. Within those fifteen hours, it turns out, she can do a lot to heal and strengthen the community.

By living directly in the community, and visiting people in their homes, a parish or community nurse knows who has enough food in the refrigerator, who needs extra help, who is struggling with money, and who needs a visit to the physician. Ellen sees much of her job as connecting people who need help with other people who want to offer help but don't know where to jump in—or are afraid of intruding on other people's privacy.

She knows who a person's friends, family, and neighbors are, and which of them might be willing to help out. She is a counselor, advocate, and educator. She helps people set up appointments, figure out questions about medications, talk through a tricky family situation, and make decisions about what the next step is. She might accompany someone to a medical appointment or coordinate with the hospital when someone is discharged from surgery. She runs flu clinics and blood pressure screenings, and sometimes teaches classes: for diabetics, new parents, and others with special concerns.

She also heads a team of volunteers that include retired physicians willing to take a look at someone's condition, and other community members willing to cook, give rides to appointments, or make home visits.

A parish or community nurse is quite different from a nurse working for the Visiting Nurse Association. VNA nurses typically are only available for short-term crisis care, and their services are generally paid for by insurance—and therefore limited by insurance coverage regulations. A community nurse, on the other hand, is generally on call most of the time, and can decide what type of care makes sense in any given situation, based on human factors, rather than corporate rules. She may, like Ellen, contract with the town (or parish) to work for a small number of total hours, but be available to work those hours at any time. Or she may simply contract to take care of the community's needs as she sees fit, for a yearly salary.

Typically community nurses are seen as part-time employees of the community or church and paid accordingly. A community or parish nurse, paid to be on call year-round, can get to know the community as a whole more deeply than a string of visiting nurses being paid by the hour.

The community nurse is generally not the one changing bandages or providing direct physical care to patients; rather, she or he works to find resources to make sure that patients can get the care, help, and company they need, playing a sort of surveillance role of watching out for people's health and well-being, getting to know everyone's individual needs, and coordinating care and resources within the community as a whole.

Any organization, neighborhood, company, or even condo association can hire a nurse to play a similar role. By offering housing—the way housing was provided for small-town school teachers and ministers—some communities or organizations may be able to reduce the already-low fees for a community nurse's care.

South Strafford, Vermont—a town with a population of about 1,000 residents—has come up with a creative solution: they simply pay their school nurse to stay for several extra hours at the end of the day, to function as a community nurse. The main difference is that she works out of the school clinic, rather than visiting people in their homes, and is only available during certain hours. Because she already knows and cares for all the children in town, however, she has a good basis for understanding the relationships and situations of many residents. Her salaried position bypasses the need for insurance, and puts profits out of the equation.

Community nursing is not for everyone. Like my home-based practice, living and working in the same community (even if you set "business hours") means that, on some level, you are always on duty. People ask your advice while waiting in line at the bank, at dinner parties, and in the school parking lot. The boundary between home and work gets blurred, and for some that can be challenging. For many, though, it is a welcome return to a more integrated way of life, and a chance to become an essential part of the commons of care.

Reduced Dependence on Technology, Increased Dependence on Each Other

We tend to imagine health care as a world of unlimited techno-logical, material, and economic resources and very *limited* social resources. For example, we expect every hospital to have all the latest equipment, yet we can't ask our neighbor to give us a ride to the hospital. We think it's normal when a doctor's visit lasts only a few minutes, yet we expect to go home from that visit with prescrip-tions for multiple medications.

As we start to understand the challenges of a failing growth economy, dwindling natural resources, supply-chain interruptions, and increasing numbers of expensive natural disasters, we might want to start looking at health care the other way around: *to under-stand that there are limits to certain material resources but plenty of untapped skills, knowledge, caring, and other social resources that we can access.* Understanding this is key as we reevaluate our whole approach to making choices in the realm of care.

Localized, human-to-human care is not only more sustainable, it is often more effective than medication or surgeries. How do we "reskill" in low-tech, human-powered medical skills to adapt to this new view? How do we change our lives to be more connected to each other?

A small local clinic may not be able to afford solar panels to run every piece of diagnostic equipment during a power outage, but the practitioners who work there can learn to be highly trained in hands-on diagnostic and treatment skills and may well get even better results. There might be fewer nursing homes in the future, but more people available to take care of each other when someone needs help. Community resources and inner resources that we never knew we had are appearing. Each neighborhood, city, state, and country has unique challenges, as well as social resources to meet those challenges.

How Sharing a Washing Machine Saved Lorraine's Life

For the first summer that the boys and I lived in the clinic, we didn't have a stove, a shower, or a washer and dryer. All those appliances had been removed when I bought the building and turned it into a multi-practitioner clinic back in 1998. My neighbor Lorraine told us that until we saved up enough money to buy new appliances, we could simply use hers.

The previous year I had treated the painful, drug-induced peripheral neuropathy that left her dragging her legs around, barely able to use a walker. I had suggested she stop taking the statin drugs that I suspected were causing the deterioration of the cholesterol-rich nerve sheaths in her legs, and encouraged her to reduce sugar, take a supplement called CoQ10, and add more grass-fed steak and butter to her diet. Her good cholesterol soared, her triglycerides dropped, her pain and weakness went away, and she was able to walk again. She might have felt she owed me a favor, but really her offer to share her home with us reflected something deeper: a working-class value of sharing resources and labor, passed down from generation to generation in her family.

Her father, Floyd, had been one of my first patients, and was the quintessential Vermonter who knew how to do everything, including raising cows and sheep on a tiny house-lot in the village by grazing them in his neighbors' backyards. He wasn't fazed by the odd manners of the wealthy "flatlanders," "trustafarians," and hippies who moved to town. He helped my Harvard-educated father-in-law buy sheep at the local auction, and helped him round them up whenever they got out. He taught me about edible weeds, and entertained my two-year-old son Henry for me when I first started seeing patients—propping him in his kitchen window to watch the dump trucks across the way.

Lorraine, at sixty-five, is much like her father: resilient. She single-handedly raised a ridiculous number of kids (some belonging to her, some belonging to a man who left her) in a trailer with no running water. She's capable of fixing a computer in the morning, editing the minister's sermon at lunchtime, talking a young person out of a suicidal depression in the afternoon, and in the evening re-caning a chair using fresh-cut cattails from the swamp next to the school. All this is somewhat surprising because she is bent over from spinal problems, has frequent dizzy spells and almost total hearing loss—all from a near-fatal bout of meningitis when she was a baby.

For years, the kids and I had already shared Lorraine's television, watching baseball games together in her living room. But now this relationship deepened. We cooked supper and ate together most nights, I took showers there when I needed to wash my hair, and I was in and out doing laundry nearly every day. In return I did a variety of favors for her: driving her to the market, picking up her mail, and giving her acupuncture in her living room.

One day, when I was there doing laundry, I noticed that she was in bed sleeping. Not unusual for her, but when I went back a few hours later she was still sleeping. I put my hand on her arm, and gently shook her. Her arm was hot, much hotter than it should have been, and she groaned when I touched her.

"Lorraine?" I said.

She groaned again. She was barely able to speak. I called her sister, and then called 911.

Lorraine ended up being hospitalized for a week. She had a bad infection and was seriously dehydrated. The doctors said that if she hadn't gotten to the hospital that day, she might well have died. That was when Lorraine and I realized the value of the arrangement we had made.

Lorraine and I together decided that I should *not* get a washer and dryer. Instead, I would keep doing laundry at her house, so that we would have the kind of regular connection that the rhythm of daily chores creates.

✄

In order to be present for other people around us, we need to have a sense that others are present for us, and that their lives are fully connected with ours, in a long-term way. Not *just* our doctors, and our spouses, but lots of people. To really settle into our own lives, we need to feel that other people will be with us through the end. No matter how disabled we become, whether or not we still recognize them, and no matter how discouraged we get, we need to feel that our people will show up and be there because we are an important part of their lives.

As we become elders, the strong connections we have with people in our community will become lifelines, ensuring that we grow old in a setting that is rich with meaning and relationships, rather than sterile, cold, and depressing. We will want to live with people we have some history with, who care about us, who like us, who have patience with our quirks, and whose children we already know, whether or not we are related to them. Knowing we are moving in this direction can also help to inspire us to take better care of ourselves now: to work on giving up addictions and emotional patterns that get in the way of having close relationships, and to work on taking care of our bodies so we can contribute to the daily chores of the household we are living in, up until the point that we can't.

≱

Lorraine has always enjoyed bartering for things. (She once convinced a famous writer to trade her large fieldstones for donuts.) But our arrangement is not just about the barter of laundry and television for my looking in on her, it's not even just about care. Our arrangement is about human contact—something Lorraine knows the value of on the deepest possible level.

When Lorraine's first child was born prematurely, the hospital told her he was not going to make it. "Well then I'm going to take him home," she said. The hospital resisted, but she was fierce. "He's my child, and I'm not going to have him die all alone in a hospital."

They gave in, and handed her the infant. She took him home and rigged up a makeshift sling that kept him right next to her skin. She hadn't read the research that shows that "marasmus" or "failure to thrive" is a life-threatening medical condition in infants that is known to be treatable by human contact. But she knew the right thing to do. She carried him around for days, and the days turned into weeks, and soon he was thriving. Fifty years later he is now one of the handsomest men around, six foot two, a strong carpenter.

Sometimes when I've had a really hard day I look across the street and see that Lorraine's light is on, and I walk over. I've come to love the dark quiet stretch of road between our two houses, late at night, long after the traffic has finally quieted down. As I walk over I can hear the distant sound of the waterfall under the covered bridge.

Lorraine is usually reading in bed. I bring in her hearing aid from the paper cup she puts it in in the kitchen at night, and hold it out. She stares at me while she puts it in and turns it on, seeing if she needs to read my lips. But I am silent. "Oh for goodness' sake," she says, when she sees my eyes welling up with tears. She pats the quilt next to her, "Get over here and tell me what happened."

I climb in next to her, start talking, and feel my body relaxing into the warmth of another human being. It is ancient and powerful medicine.

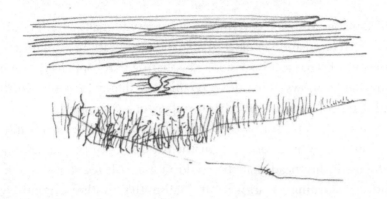

Care Banks and Home Sharing

Just after the financial crisis in 2008, a city planner named Gwen Hallsmith who lives just north of me in Montpelier, Vermont, applied for a community innovation grant from the stimulus package to set up a web-based networking system called a "Care Bank" to connect neighbors who want to share help. Based on a time-banking and barter model, Care Banks have a unique focus: building communities that enjoy caring for each other in a variety of ways.

Everyone who joins both gives and receives services, though not always with the same person. These services can take the form of companionship, rides, household assistance, healthy activities, standard or alternative health care, cooking, and more. You can bank hours whenever someone uses your services, and withdraw hours for any other service. Most importantly, all hours are valued equally. Care Banks put forth once-basic, but now "radical," notions:

- Every human being is an asset.
- Everyone matters.
- Everyone has something to offer.

Often, elders and people with disabilities are only on the *receiving* end of help. Yet a home-bound person may be the perfect person to call someone who is recovering from surgery to make sure they are okay, to remind another elder to take their medication, or to read to a person who has lost his vision. The sharing that happens through Care Banks allows everyone to retain their dignity and self-worth and share equally with all other members of a community.

Hallsmith came to this idea because of a crisis in her own family. Her mother was a brilliant mathematician—so fast at adding numbers in her head that she could race a cash register and win. Without warning, a stroke left Hallsmith's mother cognitively impaired and so paralyzed on one side that she couldn't even shift her body from her wheelchair into her bed. She wasn't eligible for assisted living because she wasn't mobile enough. Hallsmith's father took on the care of his wife, lifting, cleaning, feeding her—at an age when he himself was starting to need help. The family tried hiring caregivers, but the wages they could afford to pay for full-time care translated to poverty-level wages for the workers, and in the meantime the caregivers themselves were struggling to pay for child care.

As Hallsmith (a city planner with a master's degree in public policy) watched her parents and their caregivers struggling, she became interested in alternatives. She had been helping to plan sustainable communities for years, but this was a problem area for which she didn't have an easy answer.

She was in the midst of writing a book on local economies and local currencies. A model of alternative currency in Japan called "Caring Relationship Tickets" caught Hallsmith's attention. Each ticket (called *fureai kippu*) is equal to an hour of service helping an elder. Let's say your grandmother lives next door to me in Tokyo, and my aging mother lives in Osaka and also needs some help. I could drive *your* grandmother to her appointments, do her grocery shopping, and check in on her twice a day. Each hour that I spent doing that would give me a credit. I could use those credits to "pay" for someone else in the network to help out *my* mother, who lives 300 miles away from me. The person helping my mother might be someone in her seventies who doesn't have an aging relative, but instead saves up the credits in order to receive care when she herself is sick or in need of help.

What was of particular interest to Hallsmith was that, in surveys, people in Japan overwhelmingly said they preferred the kind of care they got in the *fureai kippu* network to the care they got from paid providers. The network attracted caregivers who were kind and well educated, and the network motivated caregivers to provide the kind of care that they would want for themselves, or for their own parents.

It was this example that inspired Hallsmith to start the Care Bank. Now Care Banks are popping up around the world as a way to organize the age-old practice of neighbors helping neighbors. Some function without any funding at all, while others raise money to cover the expenses of having staff to help coordinate and connect people who are using the web-based network to find each other.

Other networks, like Homeshare International, have sprung up that help to connect people who want to include living space in the sharing of caregiving or chores. Families that have an extra room might take in an elder or someone dealing with chronic illness in order to have someone home when the kids get back from school. An elder living alone might offer a room in their house in exchange for rides, cooking, and company. Home-share programs are like a matchmaking service, screening participants, giving advice on how to make sure you are compatible with your potential housemate or caregiver, and helping to coordinate matches between caregivers and those in need.

Adopting Each Other

As I was reading an article about gift economies, I began discussing it with my son Henry.

"It is hard to imagine living without money," he said.

I pointed out that for most of his life he *had* lived without money. Most families operate on a gift economy, where goods and services are offered without expectation of money or even barter. We give our children food, housing, clothing, shelter, health care, toys, counseling, training in various skills, transportation, and many other things simply because our children are part of our family and we love them. We often do the same for our siblings, nephews, nieces, grandchildren, and parents as we get older. Some of us do this for our friends, as well. Money is not the currency in families, friendships, and tight-knit communities. The currency is care.

My mother's mother lived to age 101. Every year, during the month of July, she and all her descendants lived together in one large house in the Adirondack Mountains. We all would help her in and out of her bath, wipe her bottom, tuck her in, cut up her food, and help her in and out of her clothes. At the same time we helped each other's babies with exactly the same processes. It seemed so easy with lots of us to help out.

Even now that she is gone, during the month of July the big kitchen is in use for hours and hours every day as brothers and sisters and cousins and friends and nieces and nephews sit and chop and stir and laugh together, all sitting down at a large table at night for our evening meal, and playing cards till the wee hours of the morning. Older children come and go from the house when they get hungry, playing outside all day. No one person does all the work; rather, when you go in the kitchen there is always something to be done, good company to do it with, and something delicious to eat while you are doing it.

If life were ideal, we'd all live close enough to keep up this money-less system of mutual care throughout the year. Unfortunately, we don't. My grandmother spent the other eleven months of her year in the nursing wing of a retirement home, cared for mostly by strangers. My brothers and sisters and I live each in our own little cubicle-like lives, thousands of miles apart, from the Yukon to

Massachusetts to New Orleans, placing high value on independence and privacy and our own life choices. [Interestingly, since I wrote that, things have changed. All of my five siblings now live near each other, two of them in the same house as my mother.]

I have learned that we can create family-like situations with the people who live around us, whether or not we are related to them.

In communities such as Amish settlements, Israeli kibbutzim, or traditional Inuit villages—where people agree to live together more or less permanently based on a shared sense of belonging—there is a similar commitment to one another's survival and well-being. They extend their view of family to a sense of community or tribe, and end up living in some version of a gift economy—sharing the work (and costs) of caring for each other. It's not just about generosity—generosity implies that one person is in a position to do a favor for another—it is also about survival. In cultures where people share work and resources, everyone benefits from care that is given to any one person, because healthy, happy people have more to give back to the whole.

Nature also operates on a gift economy. The apple tree doesn't say to the deer, "I will only give you apples if you pay me." The river doesn't say to the human, "I will only give you water if you pay me." If we extend our view of family beyond its normal bounds, to our neighborhood, and to our larger human and nonhuman community, we can actually start to imagine a moneyless economy in the realm of care.

My patient Boots and I have had an interesting arrangement for about fifteen years now. He takes care of my flower gardens and I take care of his back. No money is involved, yet it is not exactly a barter, either, because we have never kept track of hours. It is simply our relationship. Some years I get more from him, and other years he gets more from me, but it doesn't matter, because a friendship has evolved, we both enjoy talking to each other while we work, we enjoy helping each other out, and we both enjoy the labor of our own work.

As community members, we get to have relationships with each other that include the pleasurable activity of giving and receiving.

I have learned that we can create family-like situations with the people who live around us, whether or not we are related to them. Each year I bring more and more of the experience of our family rhythm in the Adirondacks into my daily life in Vermont—sharing cooking, care, play, and work with others in my community.

Even when there is money involved, one can still operate with a gift-economy mentality. Whenever a patient hands me a check, I feel as if I am receiving a gift, and I've rarely turned anyone away for lack of ability to pay. Because I operate on a sliding scale, each patient has to take a moment to think about how much the time I spent with them means to them, what it is worth to them, and how much they can afford to give me.

Once I came home and my yard was raked and the trash barrels were straightened. The hole in the driveway was filled in, and the hose I'd left out was rolled up and tucked back into place. There was a card stuck in the door from a patient saying, "I would have liked to pay you more, but since I couldn't, I brought my kids over and we had fun cleaning up your yard. We know that as a single mom there's never enough time!"

Creating Resilient Leadership among Care Providers

"There is a pervasive form of contemporary violence to which the idealist most easily succumbs: activism and overwork. The rush and pressure of modern life are a form, perhaps the most common form, of its innate violence. To allow oneself to be carried away by a multitude of conflicting concerns, to surrender to too many demands, to commit oneself to too many projects, to want to help everyone in everything, is to succumb to violence. The frenzy of our activism neutralizes our work for peace. It destroys our own

inner capacity for peace. It destroys the fruitfulness of our own
work, because it kills the root of inner wisdom which makes work
fruitful."

—**Thomas Merton**, *Conjectures of a Guilty Bystander*

Things change when a friend is struck by lightning.

Our town was remarkably resilient following Connor's death,
but I was struggling. When the sky rumbled, my heart jumped. I
woke up terrified in the mornings. Connor, just sixteen years old,
had been a close friend of Henry's, and was struck while hurrying
back from the fields at a nearby farm—trying to reach shelter from
the approaching storm.

Now the huge thunderstorms that were starting to sweep through
our neighborhood nearly every afternoon in the midsummer heat
made me nervous, and I found myself constantly shooing Henry
and Alden inside. Three generations of Connor's family were all
patients of mine, but I was in no shape to support them. I needed
time off to think and recover, but that was not an option. In the
six weeks before Connor's death, I had lost two other dear friends.
Then, just a few weeks after Connor's death, I heard on the radio
that David Rakoff, my closest male friend from college, had died of
cancer.

After the first two deaths I responded with resiliency, organiz-
ing support groups to grieve Don's suicide, and bedside vigils for
Tipi's last days. But Connor's death left me reeling, and David's
left me shocked and numb. It was less than a year after Hurricane
Irene. All of this had me worrying what things would be like when
the climate warmed up even further and the storms got even more
violent. I hadn't yet learned about soil restoration. I hadn't met any
carbon cowboys. As far as I could tell, there was no hope anywhere
on the horizon.

Without enough sleep, my mind went to dark places—I started
imagining a world where huge numbers of people were dying in
natural disasters and everyone left alive was horribly depressed. I

was supposed to take care of them all. It wasn't pretty. How was I going to care for others when I couldn't deal with my own feelings? I was not used to being the one asking for help.

Many providers become caretakers because of early (sometimes traumatic) experiences in which we needed to take care of others before we were really ready. Often these were chaotic circumstances where we weren't getting proper care ourselves, and caretaking became part of our identity before the rest of our identity was fully formed. In other cases, this identity is passed down through generations. No matter where it started, it was a survival tactic—"If I take care of the people around me, then I will stand a good chance of getting what I need"—and it worked. This type of early experience can set us up to take wretched care of ourselves, even while we are providing excellent care for others. Some of us become so used to running on adrenalin that we function brilliantly during emergencies, but then collapse later on.

Under normal circumstances, the body moves back and forth between activation and regulation, sympathetic and parasympathetic responses to the circumstances around us. When we are startled by a sudden loud noise, for example, the body shifts briefly into "fight, flight, or freeze" mode. Rational thought (in the frontal lobe) briefly shuts down, and instincts (in the amygdala) take over. The heart races as it gears up to run. Sleep and digestion are put on hold, until the body is sure that the danger is over. Then, under normal circumstances, it relaxes and settles back down into its usual "rest and digest" mode. Rational thinking returns: "Oh, it was just the cat, knocking over the lamp."[3]

As I struggled with the untimely deaths of four friends in three months, and a rapidly unraveling climate, I knew that trauma is not linear; it is cumulative and compounding. If there isn't enough time to process things, or if sleep is interrupted for too many nights, two drops of adrenalin become four, and four drops of adrenalin become

---

3   See psychologist Peter Levine's work, in particular *In an Unspoken Voice: How the Body Heals Trauma and Restores Goodness* (Berkeley: North Atlantic Books, 2010).

eight, and before you know it, there is a flood. Things might look fine, and then suddenly a person's system gets overloaded and goes into "dorsal vagal shutdown," a longer term "freeze" mode where our reptilian brain hijacks the whole system and refuses to shut off, like a car with the accelerator pedal stuck to the floor.

It's not unlike the way a climate that has been gradually shifting suddenly spirals out of control as icebergs melt and forests catch fire, pouring unexpected additional carbon into the atmosphere. It's not unlike the way oil prices suddenly spiral upward, or the way economies collapse under compounding debt.

Yet I also knew that that same principle applies to positive change. Small fruitful actions can start to build, without anyone noticing. You might think no one cares about an oil pipeline, and then one day thousands of people link hands and surround the White House, in protest. Just when nature seems to have been completely forgotten, a country like Bolivia votes to include the rights of nature in their new constitution. And one morning you wake up and hear that people in Detroit are raising sheep in the city streets, and planting organic gardens in the empty backyards of homes that were abandoned during the housing crisis.

Hope is a discipline, and even though I felt beaten down, I was not giving up.

I harnessed my adrenalin to fight back against my own fear and discouragement, using the same dark humor I had shared with David in college. "There are still a few billion people left in the world for you to be close to," I told myself "You probably won't end up ALL alone." I pushed myself to lean heavily on friends and family, and show them what a wreck I was, even though it felt dangerous.

I made everyone around me promise that they wouldn't kill themselves, no matter how hard their lives got. ("Oh I'd never do that," said my friend Bob, the software engineer, who had also lost a friend to suicide. "If it got really bad I would just parachute naked into another country.")

It took many months, but gradually I got back on my feet. I started to apply the same principles to my life that I was suggesting for our health-care system: simple, local, scaled down. I started to think about becoming sturdy and dependable for myself, rather than being inspiring for others. This meant taking a break for lunch, doing the dishes, and picking up my clothes from the floor, rather than joining more committees or taking on more patients. I knew I could not continue to take care of everyone around me, or fight every fight alone. I needed my life to be more like a relay race and less like a marathon.

Other people I knew were feeling similarly. I had been going for walks with another single mother, Vanessa, who worked full time as a climate-change activist. She talked to me about how her fellow activists were getting burned out and forgetting to take care of themselves, and how it was impacting their ability to be effective. Our local minister, Tom, was working more than full time looking out for people in our community, while being paid a part-time salary, and he was considering leaving his job. My friend Rebecca, a trauma psychologist, was thinking about closing her practice because she needed to take better care of herself. Abby, who ran the local women's shelter, was feeling exasperated and overworked because grant money was running low and funding for projects was being cut just as the harsh new economy was leaving more women homeless.

I sat down with my friend Mark Kutolowski—an oblate of the Benedictine Christian community, a primitive skills teacher, and a wilderness guide—to figure out what to do next.

Mark and I had met a few years before, when I had taken my boys to a class he was teaching on how to start fires without matches. We became fast friends after we realized we both had a love for God, for unpasteurized heavy cream, and for jumping in cold rivers. He taught me about contemplative prayer, and I taught him the principles of effective peer support. He taught me how to butcher a deer and find wild edibles, and I taught him the concepts of traditional Chinese medicine, and how to cook venison stew.

As a deeply spiritual community member, to whom many people turned for free and unlimited counseling, Mark was struggling with some of the same feelings of burnout.

Instead of trying to help everyone, we wanted to find specific leverage points where the knowledge and skills we already had could do the most good. It seemed to us that the best way to do that was to support those working toward change, to make sure that they didn't get burned out the way we were, while also creating a larger community of practice that would support all of us in taking better care of ourselves, based on the peer-coaching model we were already using with each other and several other friends.

We started piecing together a curriculum in mutual support, deep self-care, and resilient leadership that was broadly applicable, easy to teach, and could be passed along safely. Then we invited a group of people to join the class. We chose people who, if they understood the principles we taught, would impact many other people's lives, including our own. We knew, from our own experience, that no matter how good a health-care or mental health system is, there is no form of medicine that can substitute for a warm, healthy community.

In our first ten-week course we had twenty participants, ranging in age from sixteen to seventy. They included hospice workers, teachers, environmental leaders, health-care providers, youth advocacy workers, farmers, and the director of the local women's shelter. Connor's sister, mother, and grandmother all ended up in our group of twenty.

We helped them to understand the role of traditional diets, as well as the history of food in the growth economy and its relationship to current health problems. We taught scientific and traditional understandings of the benefits of meditation and we provided support in developing a daily contemplative practice. We gave them tools for understanding and overcoming addictions, support in developing a relationship with the natural world, and a simple, efficient exercise routine. Most importantly, we included skills for building peer-support networks, and addressed the challenges of stepping forward into leadership.

On the final weekend of our course, we spent two full days together. We started each morning with exercise outside, followed by a leap into the river where we stood around talking in our under-gitchies. We lay in the sun looking at catfish under the footbridge, then shared stories of our lives. We cooked fantastic nutrient-dense lunches with rich discussions about the benefits of broths, mushrooms, and wild edibles as we feasted. We had long, deep conversations about how our economic system affected our health, and how we might work together to effect change in the larger system. We ended each day with a quiet meditation. Both days were soft and delicious sunny spring weather and we spent most of our time outside. It felt, to all of us, like the first two days of a newly made world.

Since then we have adapted parts of the Health, Empowerment, And Resiliency Training (HEART) course to broaden its impact. Between the two of us, we've worked with groups of ministers, climate change leaders, college students, hospital food service managers (at Diane Imrie's "Healthy Food for Health Care" retreats), and 250 children at our local elementary school. Our students, in turn, have passed the course material on to military veterans at the VA hospital, to high school and college students, and beyond, while we all continue to broaden our networks of support.

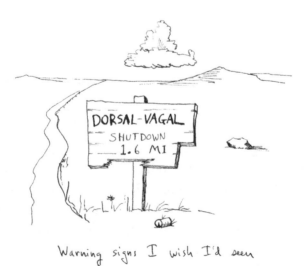

Warning signs I wish I'd seen

CHAPTER TEN

Universal Health Care As If the Whole Universe Mattered

"Our 'Western' medical system is itself but a compendium of knowledge, wisdom and therapeutics accumulated from past cultures and societies from around the world. We should be justifiably proud of the accomplishments of medical science, but at the same time not lose perspective that these advancements, in many cases, emerged only in the past half-century. My point is that we should not be so quick to sever the umbilical cord of our medical system from the womb of the last remaining cultures that helped give it birth. We do so at our great loss."

—Christopher Herndon[1]

The ancient texts of Chinese medicine describe blood and vital oxygen (*"Qi"*) moving through an inner landscape in which they fill up wells, trickle out of springs, move into streams, pour into rivers, and flow into oceans. Those flows can be influenced by acupuncture needles, carefully placed, which function like rocks in moving water to divert or enhance flows in certain areas. Illnesses are associated with seasons and elements, and treated not only with acupuncture but also with herbs, minerals, and other natural

---

1   Rhett A. Butler, "How Rainforest Shamans Treat Disease," Mongabay, November 10, 2009, http://news.mongabay.com/2009/1110-herndon_amazon_shaman. html; and Christopher N Herndon, et al., "Disease Concepts and Treatment by Tribal Healers of an Amazonian Forest Culture," *Journal of Ethnobiology and Ethnomedicine* 27, no. 5 (2009).

substances that clear excess heat, moisten dryness, extinguish wind, and drain dampness.

Traditional forms of medicine see the body as a reflection of the natural world, and use natural means to treat it. In Ayurvedic medicine from India—which classifies patients' constitutions and symptoms according to their balance of air, fire, earth, and water—food and herbs are used to correct imbalances in these elements. Islamic physicians had a similar system.

The practice of ecological, pattern-based medicine was not limited to the East. Ancient Greek and Roman physicians classified illnesses in similar ways, and Hildegard of Bingen—a twelfth-century herbalist, writer, composer, and mystic who was also the abbess of a Benedictine monastery and hospital in Germany—wrote of the need to approach the body as a garden.[2]

By the time I entered acupuncture school in 1990, some of the more ecological aspects of the practice of Chinese medicine had already been stripped away, influenced by the spread of modern Western medical science. We learned only the barest details of the ecological view of the body, enough to leave us hungry and searching for more details—what was the difference between points classified as "rivers" versus "streams"? Why were some points classified as "windows of the sky"? Our teachers, trained during the Cultural Revolution in China, could only answer us in very broad terms.

In our textbooks from China, the highly descriptive point names (like *spirit waste land* and *essential dew*) had been replaced with numbers (*Kidney 1, Kidney 2, Kidney 3*). We had to find other books in order to study the poetic names, but we could only guess at their deeper meanings until teachers who had held on to the traditional knowledge began to surface, years later.[3] In school I

2   Victoria Sweet, *God's Hotel: A Doctor, a Hospital, and a Pilgrimage to the Heart of Medicine* (New York: Riverhead Books, 2012).
3   The Taoist principles underlying the ecological theories of acupuncture would not surface in most schools in the United States until after I graduated, when teachers like Jeffrey Yuen, an 88th-generation Taoist master, decided to share their knowledge and restore the spiritual and environmental roots of Chinese medicine. (Yuen has

learned to locate points by measurement, using Western anatomical landmarks (e.g., *three body inches distal to the head of the fibula*) until I was able to find blind Japanese practitioners who were willing to teach me a more accurate form of point location based on touch and sensory cues in our fingertips *(slightly moist, with a very slight raised area around it—as if you were feeling between the lips of a very small dog).*

But even though our formal education only hinted at the depth of the Chinese traditions, I did learn other useful things, direct benefits from the scientific method. I got to explore the literal inner landscape of the body in the cadaver anatomy lab, seeing sliced-open layers of the body that would have been forbidden to most ancient medical practitioners. I got to learn about biochemical and physiological processes that make digestion possible, and electrical pathways that carry nerve signals from our brains to our limbs and back again, allowing us to walk and talk. I got to work with Parkinson's patients and see what happens when one chemical goes awry, and I got to work with some of the very first AIDS patients and see what happens when a virus causes the immune system to stop functioning.

I came away from my education with a variety of ways to look at the body and the world, all interesting, all valid in their own ways. I loved all these aspects, and I integrated them into my practice, where I easily switch between—and often combine—a modern biomedical view and a traditional ecological view.

It's this perspective that got me thinking about the parallels between what's been happening in the health of our inner landscapes as our outer landscapes shift—even more so as I began examining the circular relationships between soil health, climate, and the health of humans and other species.

---

kept transcribers busy for years filling volume after volume with his oral transmission of the tradition.)

Correlations between Human
and Planetary Conditions

Whether we like the idea of it or not, the microbial life inside us and around us is the intelligence behind our earthly and bodily immune systems, the energy that keeps things in a dynamic flow, and the glue that holds things, literally, together. The microorganisms in our soil and in our intestines exude the mucosal slimes that keep our soils intact and our digestive tracts healthy. It's no coincidence that the digestive system is called the "earth" element in Chinese medicine.

Perhaps the greatest challenge to our human and planetary health is the result of a thinning of the microbiologically rich (and therefore) "mucosal" layer in our guts and in our soils, creating, in both cases, a leakage problem and an inflammatory response in the larger system.

The overuse of antibiotics in medicine and in our food-stream kills off important bacteria in our guts. When we lose the bacterially rich, slimy mucosal layer of our guts, our intestines become too permeable, leading to interior leakage in which food particles and toxins get absorbed into the bloodstream, creating an inflammatory response.

Modern agricultural practices create a thinning of the microorganism-rich mucosal layer of topsoil, leaching off nutrients and pollutants into the streams, rivers, and oceans as they flow through the body of the earth—not unlike the leaky gut syndrome. The loss of microorganisms in soils, and the resulting loss of soil's carbon- and moisture-holding capacity, has created an "inflammatory" response in the global climate and local ecosystems.

In cancer, I find another parallel between our inner and outer worlds. Cancer is unrestricted growth—or a failure of the regulation of growth—not unlike what we see in our global economy. Cancer cells are normal cells gone awry: their only problem is that they take up more than their fair share of space, and use up more resources than they should. This unrestricted growth can be due to "too much self-sufficiency" in regulating their own behavior, an insensitivity to antigrowth signals, or an evasion of other limiting factors.[4] When cancerous cells metastasize, or colonize a new area, they do so by diverting the blood supply from other tissues, so they can use the food, water, and fuel in the blood for their own self-serving new lifestyle.[5]

Sound familiar? Cancer is eerily similar to the processes we've seen of unlimited economic growth and colonization in a global economy, in which a small percent of the population places its own interests above the survival of the whole, ignoring warning signs, evading attempts to limit growth, and using up more than its fair share of what should be commonly shared resources.

Disconnection is at the heart of modern illness.

The Wisdom Tradition

> "For in her is a spirit intelligent, holy, unique, manifold, subtle, agile, clear . . . kindly, firm, secure, tranquil, all-powerful, all seeing, and pervading all spirits . . . For Wisdom is mobile beyond all motion, and she penetrates and pervades all things by reason of her purity . . . For she is the refulgence of eternal light, the spotless mirror of the power of Love, the image of God's goodness, and she, who is one, can do all things, while herself perduring."
>
> —Wisdom 7:22b-8:1

For several hundred years, both science and religion in Western culture have seen humanity as something quite separate from, and superior to, the rest of nature. (Read the introduction to almost

4 D. Hanahan and R. A. Weinberg, "Hallmarks of Cancer: The Next Generation," *Cell*, 2011 Mar 4;144(5):646–74.
5 Priscilla LeMone, et al., *Medical Surgical Nursing* (Pearson, 2011), 389.

any philosophical, spiritual, or scientific book written by a white man in the past two centuries and you will likely find a line that lauds humanity's unique capacity for consciousness, intelligence, or spirituality.)

Along with that attitude came a belief that certain people were also superior to others, and could therefore take more than their fair share of power and resources in order to survive. During that brief nap in our consciousness, a few dangerous ideas settled into our world view:

- Success in medicine and agriculture involves experimenting on and triumphing over nature, rather than aligning ourselves with the cycles and patterns of nature in order to thrive
- People living in "primitive" cultures have little to teach us, and need to be educated out of their backward ways in order to be healthy and happy[6]
- Medicine and agriculture are highly profitable businesses, rather than collaborative community responsibilities

We are waking up to a world that is almost unrecognizable to our souls and our cells.

How do we remember what we have forgotten?

Most or all world religions have a lesser-known "wisdom" tradition. These traditions teach a "unitive" path that sees and values the connectedness of the whole. Often based on meditation and mindfulness, wisdom practices give rise to non-hierarchical ways of seeing the world, in which one recognizes that everything is a small

6   Indigenous cultures tended to have long, healthy lifespans before they came in contact with the food, cities, toxic waste, and pathogens—unfamiliar to their immune systems—that came along with colonization, global capitalism, and industrialization. See Weston A. Price, *Nutrition and Physical Degeneration* (La Mesa: Price-Pottenger Nutrition Foundation, 2008).

Strengthening Connections:
How Mindfulness Changes the Brain[*,†]

A regular practice of mindfulness:

- Increases the size of the brain regions that are related to attention and sensory processing
- Increases the brain's capacity to detect emotional cues from other people
- Increases the immune system's production of antibodies, which protect against disease
- Decreases levels of the stress hormone called cortisol, helping the body to relax
- Decreases anxiety, depression, and anger
- Helps people to manage physical pain

Students who go through a mindfulness training program:

- Show improved academic performance
- Feel more relaxed when taking tests
- Are calmer and less aggressive with each other
- Sleep more soundly
- Are more focused

Parents who practice mindfulness describe:

- Increased satisfaction with their parenting
- More social interactions with their children
- Less stress
- More closeness as a couple

[*] Excerpted from Greg Flaxman and Lisa Flook, "A Brief Summary of Mindfulness Research," accessed June 9, 2015, http://marc.ucla.edu/ workfiles/pdfs/MARC-mindfulness-research-summary.pdf.

[†] F. Zeidan, et al., "Mindfulness Meditation-Related Pain Relief: Evidence for Unique Brain Mechanisms in the Regulation of Pain," *Neuroscience Letters* 520, no. 2 (2012):165–73.

but important part of the whole, and at the same time, each part is an all-important microcosm, reflecting the elegance and intelligence of the whole. There is a sense, in the wisdom traditions, of the sacred whole permeating everything, and of everything being sacred in and of itself.

These practices (taught in Sufism, Contemplative Christianity, Taoism, Tibetan Buddhism, Native Earth-based Spirituality, and Kabbala) have often been overshadowed by the more dualistic (good versus evil) and hierarchical forms of each religion. But in recent decades, the wisdom traditions and their contemplative practices have begun to resurface.

Recent neuroscience shows that the contemplative, meditative practices used by these traditions can literally reconnect parts of the brain—healing us from the tearing apart that happened under the dualistic paradigm—while increasing the size of the brain regions related to focus, sensory processing, and empathy. There is a resulting shift in perception—toward curiosity and presence, rather than endless categorizing and critique.

If our modern illnesses are related to an increasing sense and experience of disconnection, then it is not surprising that contemplative practices—with their ability to reconnect us to our senses, our surroundings, and our neighbors—also help the immune system, decrease stress hormones, improve sleep, and reduce physical pain.[7,8] The work of creating health is the work of restoring connection.

The stories of the wisdom traditions often reflect three phases in the evolution of human consciousness. These are simultaneously the phases of a well-lived human life, as well as phases and cycles in human history:

7   Greg Flaxman and Lisa Flook, "A Brief Summary of Mindfulness Research," accessed June 9, 2015, http://marc.ucla.edu/workfiles/pdfs/MARC-mindfulness-research-summary.pdf.
8   F. Zeidan, et al., "Mindfulness Meditation-Related Pain Relief: Evidence for Unique Brain Mechanisms in the Regulation of Pain," *Neuroscience Letters* 520, no. 2 (2012):165–73.

- In the first phase, we intuitively understand that we are part of the whole without having to question it, or even think about it. In this phase we live in a unitive consciousness, like the rest of nature, within the flows and patterns of the whole ecological system.[9]
- In the middle, so-called rational phase (reductionism), we see ourselves as separate from the whole. We see some people/animals/processes/parts of the body as good, and others as evil. We rely entirely on our huge, rational forebrain and forget that we are part of the whole.[10]
- In the third stage, the "post-rational" stage, we again enter unitive consciousness, but from a place that knows the pain of separation. We choose to see ourselves, and act, as part of the whole, because we have experienced, and now understand, the problems of disconnection.[11]

If we look at these stages as three historical stages in our society's relationship to nature, we are just beginning to enter the third stage. We now know, without a doubt (having used our large brains, microscopes, and scientific analyses to "prove" it), that we cannot thrive or even survive without cooperating with our inner and outer companions: from our neighbors, to our gut bacteria, to the phytoplankton in the oceans. We know that we live within an ecosystem and that an ecosystem lives within us, and that every living thing is a reservoir of sacred genetic information—a record of adaptation and resiliency, compiled since the beginning of creation, and continuing to create our world in the present moment.

9   In the Christian tradition this is "the Garden of Eden."
10   When we "ate from the tree of knowledge," to use a Christian metaphor.
11   In Christian terms this is "the Realm of God." Jesus's frequent admonition to "Repent, for the Kingdom of Heaven is at hand" is not a doomsday proposition, as is commonly supposed. Nor is he asking people to feel badly about themselves. Rather, this phrase is more aptly translated as *"Look from a larger perspective. Everything around you is sacred."* The word translated as "Repent" is actually the Greek word *Meta-noia*: "larger knowing" or "beyond the intellect," which completely changes the second half of the sentence.

To treat ourselves and our illnesses in the postindustrial era, we will need to extend our view of "universal health care" to include the "universe" of our entire planet. We will also need to re-imagine care itself. For thousands of years we have been asked by native and contemplative traditions to broaden our view. The time has come for us to care for the mycorrhizal fungi and honeybees, not just because they help to produce our food, but because they are part of our community, and part of our own larger body. We can respect their wisdom and look out for their well-being, the way a neighbor cares for a neighbor, the way a community supports its teachers, the way our hands spend time washing and caring for themselves, but also the rest of the body—our toes, our legs, our ears—because it is all one body.

Given that we haven't even agreed whether universal health care is something we want for all humans, it may be a leap to ask people to consider extending universal health care to frogs and seals, to rivers and oceans, and even to microscopic organisms. But it is essential. The natural world is actually part of our health-care system—an intelligent and experienced provider, and worthy itself of deep care.

Wild Law

> "We went to Geneva, the six nations, the great Lakota nation
> . . . and the indigenous people said 'What of the rights of the
> natural world? Where is the seat for the Buffalo or the Eagle?
> Who is speaking for the waters of the earth? Who is speaking
> for the trees and the forests? Who is speaking for the Fish, for
> the Whales, for the Beavers, for our children?'"[12]

In 2012, a neighbor and I gathered signatures to introduce a vote in our town on the question of whether our state should consider protecting the rights of nature under the law.

---

12 Oren Lyons, "Our Mother Earth," *Parabola* 6, no. 1 (1984):91–93, quoted in
Gregory Cajete, *Look to the Mountain: An Ecology of Indigenous Education* (Durango:
Kivakí Press, 1994).

This type of legislation had already become law in certain US towns and cities, and in 2008 was incorporated into the constitution of the entire country of Ecuador. Bolivia has done the same. Under these new laws, the ecosystem itself—or any part of it, such as a river, forest, or species—can now be named as the defendant.[13] People still have rights to use natural systems in ways that do no long-term harm, and courts help to weigh the proper balance between humans' legal rights (as members of the natural world), the rights of nature itself, and the interdependence between the two. But, rather than treating nature as property under the law, these laws acknowledge that nature in all its life-forms has the *"right to exist, persist, maintain and regenerate its vital cycles."*

In Ecuador, this legal defense has already been used to help efforts to protect the Amazonian rain forest as mitigation against climate change, to stop illegal mining, and repair damage to local waterways.

South African attorney Cormac Cullinan's book *Wild Law: A Manifesto for Earth Justice*[14] explores the ins and outs of giving nature legal rights of its own, and comes out strongly in favor of it.

Here is how I understand it: The lines between our own health and the health of our ecosystems are much blurrier than we thought they were when our current environmental legislation was written— we didn't understand about the interwoven relationships between soil and water, or pesticides and pollinators. We didn't understand the deep connection between our ecosystems and our own mental and physical health.

Current environmental legislation falls under the "commerce" clause of the US Constitution. These laws view nature as property, and mainly serve to preserve one person's commercial interests against another's by regulating how much damage can reasonably be done, and how much of nature can be used up. When legal damages

---

13 Peter D. Burdon, "Wild Law, the Philosophy of Earth Jurisprudence," *Alternative Law Journal* 35, no. 2 (2010).

14 Cormac Cullinan, *Wild Law: A Manifesto for Earth Justice* (White River Junction, VT: Chelsea Green, 2011), 47–49.

are awarded, they are given from one person to another to make up for the money that has been lost because of the damage that was done to natural property. (This has been compared to previous laws entitling a slave owner to damages when another person beat or killed his slave.) When nature has no rights, and no person can claim damages, there are many situations where there is no lawsuit possible.

Even when *citizens'* rights are protected in an environmental lawsuit, nature itself is often not. For example, under current laws, if a person wins a lawsuit against a hydrofracking operation that polluted his or her drinking water, the money awarded by the courts would not go to restore the polluted aquifer. Instead, the money would be used to pay the person for the trouble of moving somewhere where there is clean water. This way of viewing nature—as something we own and can replace or buy more of if we need to—does not reflect the reality that we live on a relatively small planet, and that we would actually need another half a planet in addition to our own in order to keep feeding our extractive appetite for natural resources. Unfortunately, paying another person rarely remediates a damaged and "used up" environment.

This is complicated even further by our current legal situation in which corporations are considered "persons" under the law. Environmental regulation can be argued to "impinge on the rights of" corporations—giving corporations legal standing to undo environmental regulation. This is particularly problematic because corporations are often capable of damaging natural systems much faster than individuals.

This can be remedied by giving nature legal standing, and giving people the right to petition on behalf of nature. New systems of health-care legislation may want to consider a similar path of understanding—including the natural world as both patient and provider, and giving nature the privileges and protections it deserves for both of those roles. Our new understanding of the interconnectedness of environmental and human health calls for updated laws that actually protect the natural systems, processes, and genetic patterns that all our current species depend on for life.

In many towns, the "Rights of Nature" article has passed. In my own town, it lost by a single vote, which drove home the importance of showing up in a democracy.

Look Before You Leap: The Precautionary Principle

Another tactic that some countries and organizations have adopted is the "precautionary principle,"[15] which states that if an action or policy has a suspected risk of causing harm to the public or to the environment, the active party (the person or company that is proposing the action) needs to prove that it is safe, rather than it being the victim's responsibility to prove that it is harmful.

The European Union has adopted this principle as a statutory requirement in their legal system, which allows policy makers to delay action or decision making in situations where there is the possibility of harm from taking a particular course or when extensive scientific knowledge on a proposal is lacking.

Policy makers and corporations therefore have a social responsibility to protect the public from exposure to harm when scientific investigation has found a plausible risk, even before all the evidence is in. These protections can be relaxed only if further scientific findings emerge that provide sound evidence that no harm will result. The precautionary principle is particularly concerned with issues that involve the impact of human actions on complex systems—such as ecosystems, living organisms, and human health—that often respond in unpredictable ways when new elements are introduced.[16]

15 "Precautionary Principle—FAQs," Science and Environmental Health Network, last modified August 5, 2015, accessed June 9, 2015, http://www.sehn.org/ppfaqs.html.
16 Sarah Catherine Walpole, Kumanan Rasanathan, and Diarmid Campbell-Lendrum, "Natural and Unnatural Synergies: Climate Change Policy and Health Equity," *Bulletin of the World Health Organization* 87 (2009):799–801.

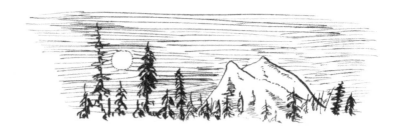

Jumping Back Into the River

"A human being is part of the whole called by us 'the universe,' a part limited in time and space. He experiences himself, his thoughts and feelings, as something separate from the rest—a kind of optical delusion of his consciousness. The striving to free oneself from this delusion is in the one issue of true religion. Not to nourish the delusion but to try to overcome it is the way to reach the attainable measure of peace of mind."

—**Albert Einstein**[17]

Every day I jump into the Ompompanoosuc River, whether it is cold and cloudy, or warm and sunny. It is my morning prayer, my baptism to start each day anew, and my cold-immersion therapy to keep my immune system strong. Sometimes there is a sign up saying that there is a high bacterial count, and that swimming is not recommended. After it rains, the water is cloudy with silt—and probably some manure coming from farms upriver. It's likely that acid rain, spraying for mosquitoes, pharmaceuticals, and gasoline spills subtly work their way into my morning dip, even when the water is clear. Sometimes I pause, and wonder if it is a good idea. But almost always, I still choose to plunge my body into the river.

Ultimately all these things will affect me whether I choose to swim directly in them or not. If the river is unhealthy, I am

---

17 Albert Einstein, Personal letter to Robert S. Marcus, on the passing of his son from polio. *The Liberator Magazine*, http://weblog.liberatormagazine.com/2010/10/einstein-on-being-human-sayings.html.

unhealthy too. I share in its troubles whether I want to or not, because I live in the same landscape.

More and more, however, I feel that I *want* to share in the river's life. I stay when a hurricane sweeps through my town, or when an emotional storm sweeps through my children's lives; why shouldn't I stay with my river and its watershed? The longer I live here, the more I see myself, my river, and all the land, streams, and animals that feed into, and are fed by, the river as one body and one whole interconnected life.

⚹

Today as I swim, I think of the millions of life-forms that are in each droplet of the water, running down my arms and forming tiny sparkling horizons, like small clear skies, as I pull myself back up onto the rocks.

My "baptism" is quite literal. I leave my human-created world, and immerse myself once again in the creation—the microorganisms— that I evolved with and from, and that are still changing along with me and inside of me. Phoebe, my small dog, partakes in her own communion, digging deep into the roots of a tree and gulping down mouthfuls of soil, full of more microorganisms in each mouthful than there are humans on Earth. She is literally eating the body of creation, and replenishing her own inner world with new life.

I close my eyes and feel the source of life pouring itself through the world. Like the waterfall near me, it is huge, thundering, endlessly flowing. All of life, in turn, pours itself back to the source in gratitude, from the manifest to the unmanifest, and around again, like the huge water-wheel that used to turn just up the river from here, creating power from power itself.

The Earth really is like that, I think to myself: The whole Earth and atmosphere pours forth health and nourishment toward all its inhabitants. And all who live here, from single-celled organisms, to plants, to the sheep up the hill from me, pour back nourishment toward the whole, each in their own way.

I know, though, that something is broken in this cycle. Since the industrial period began, we humans have continued to take from the whole but have given back less and less. We have drained the Earth's resources without replenishing them, and increasingly without even expressing gratitude. We have lost track of the fact that our existence, our health, and even our consciousness itself, is inextricably mixed with our environment. The glaciers melt. The oceans rise. The waterwheel wobbles and spits back gray water into the clear waterfall. Power is out of balance.

⊿

I sit on the rock, feeling the comforting sensation of my body readjusting itself to the pull of the larger magnetic field of the Earth, and a jewel-wing damsel fly settles onto my knee. He opens and closes four black velvet wings above his shimmering blue-green body in time with my own breathing. I am stunned by his beauty. When he takes flight, my eyes drift to the water bugs jumping among the river's slow swirl of bubbles, creating ancient patterns that remind my brain of dances far older than any I have learned in this lifetime.

Smaller life-forms have at least one huge advantage over us: they evolve and adapt far more quickly than we do—therefore they are hugely resilient. They have learned to work together and to regulate their own behavior in order to keep the environment around them relatively stable, so they can survive. What can we learn from them?

Life itself has evolved from a more linear stage—in which cells, working on their own, created the same structures over and over again—to a new stage wherein two cells could miraculously meet, open their tightly held boundaries, and exchange the gifts of their ancient genetic codes to make new, uniquely differing, and more resilient individuals. If single-celled organisms can do this in order to solve problems, then so—I believe—can we.

Respect for Our Inner Working Class.
The microorganisms that we host in our bodies do much of the work that we take credit for. They carry out and direct many of the

essential processes that enable us to think, play, and work in daily life. Even the cells that we call our own—that make up the brain, heart, eyes, ears—are in fact microorganisms that have organized themselves, through an ongoing process of creation (also called evolution) to work together in a living system that we call "a human body."[18] You could call it a workers' cooperative.

Society teaches us to credit the "owners" and "managers" of companies with the products of a company's labor—not the working-class people who sit in the factory and do the real work. When we don't understand the role of microorganisms in our bodies, and try to take too much control, we disrespect the wisdom and inherent power of our own inner working class, and we make management decisions that tend to lead to poor functioning of the whole. Repairs aren't made, morale is low, and—as short-term solutions are offered in the form of drugs—the "workers" are less empowered to take responsibility for getting their job done. Our human–microbe collaborative system ends up with low energy levels, unstable emotions, poor immune function, and other problems.

Microorganisms in the soil also do important work that we are mostly unaware of, because—again, like the working class—their work is quiet and hidden from view. Yet these workers provide most of the essential goods and services we rely on for daily life: making nutrients available to plants (and animals that eat the plants), filtering out toxins, regulating the flow and storage of water, allowing plants to grow and thereby produce oxygen, and influencing our weather and climate. They also create the stable structural conditions (in what would otherwise be the shifting sands and water) of the Earth's surface that make it possible for us to build houses and roads that don't collapse or wash away. Land managers who don't recognize the role or value of soil microorganisms end up creating conditions in which those organisms cannot do their work or even survive— exposing them to unnecessary "occupational hazards" with agricul-

18 Lynn Margulis and Dorion Sagan, *Acquiring Genomes: A Theory of the Origins of Species* (Perseus Books Group, 2002).

tural machinery, life-threatening temperatures through tillage and bare soil, over- and undergrazing, and dousing with chemicals.

The microorganisms in the ocean—though I've focused on them less, because we tend to manage them less (but with the advent of geoengineering, that is quickly changing)—created most of the oxygen that made life on Earth possible, and continue to produce more than half of all of the oxygen we breathe.

When we *do* value the quiet work that is going on inside and around us, we are far more likely to make decisions that create healthy working conditions for the microorganisms in our inner and outer landscapes. The essence of life is that organisms naturally tend to work together in *self-organizing* systems, where they solve problems and evolve in creative ways, without external control or constant intervention. This is true on many scales. Yet in our ways of managing society, bodies, and land, we constantly try to control and regulate the creative processes around us, to *make* those self-organizing groups do things, instead of *letting* them.

We could claim our own place as workers: full participants, not "owners," working side by side with all other organisms in the powerful work of restoration. That will entail a wholesale shift in our thought processes as a society. But until that point, as individual "stewards" our management strategies (of our land and bodies) should be supportive, respectful, and mostly hands off.

Our world, both inside and out, continues to be shaped by organisms we can't even see. Gut bacteria influence our inner weather—our behavior, moods, and health. Other microorganisms influence our outer weather—phytoplankton in the ocean help to regulate the temperature and oxygen concentration on the planet; soil microorganisms, working in concert with plants and fungi, shuttle atmospheric carbon back into deep storage in the earth, and bacteria that ride around in clouds help raindrops and snowflakes to form.[19]

If we are willing to collaborate with them, and learn to let them lead the dance, it's possible that their superior ability to change and

19 Brent C. Christner, "Cloudy with a Chance of Microbes," *Microbe* 7, no 2 (2012).

regulate may contribute solutions to the problems we are facing—but only if we can listen to their wisdom and support them in their silent work.

※

The solutions are there. Sometimes it's just hard to see them.

That's because the solutions—to the problems we have created in our profit-driven industrial lives—are hidden in the places that we have disconnected from. As the pesky parts of nature, microorganisms, "inconvenient" people, and traditional cultures have been stamped out or pushed to the margins, we have lost sight of the lessons they carried with them. We unintentionally disconnected our lives from the natural systems and interspecies relationships we have always relied on for health, as well as from the cultural traditions and wisdom of the resilient people who have learned how to survive during difficult circumstances. We have done this just at the point when we are likely to need them the most.

The truth is, in the rush toward progress, we have lost a lot. So what do we do?

We can choose to welcome in, befriend, and learn from the people and places we forgot: the good bacteria in our bellies struggling to survive our modern diets; the soil microorganisms struggling to survive our modern agriculture; the medicinal herbs growing as "weeds" at the edges of our sidewalks; the elders hidden away in the nursing home down the street; the children and adults who question convention, learn differently, or don't follow social rules; poor people and communities that have survived catastrophes; and the indigenous cultures around the world that have been pushed aside to make room for "progress"—all of these could be helping us to come up with elegant solutions to the problems at hand.

Health care, if we do it right, will have gone full circle—from early healers practicing in isolated locales, to specialists practicing high-tech medicine on a global scale, to a new era in which we are called to practice collaborative, whole-systems care—taking into account local communities and global concerns, while welcoming the perspectives that come from the microscope, the telescope, the curious child, and communion with the world itself.

The elements and forces that first formed our planet continue to unfold within us and around us. They connect us back through the eons, forward into the future, and across continents and species.

When we can stand in the center and look at the whole, we can understand issues that once perplexed us. Healing the old rifts between science and religion, between humans and nature, between old wisdom and new discoveries, is a matter of becoming more and more aware of our common source. True health care, as we move forward, will trust the intelligence of the whole.

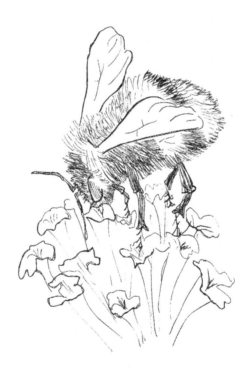

EPILOGUE

As I walk over to Patrick at the baseball game, I have no idea how this conversation is going to go, and I'm a little surprised that I am risking it.

Patrick and his business partner grew up here in Thetford, and now own the beautiful dairy farm in the eastern end of town, known at one time for its milk-scrounging cats—perhaps 100 of them—that moved in waves, in perfect unison, like a flock of birds. For many years, the cats were uncatchable, and so they kept breeding, but now they have dwindled in number to a modest posse. The farm, perched in the hills and spreading down into the floodplain along the Connecticut River, belonged to Lorraine's brother-in-law before he retired. It's a substantial portion of the agricultural land in our town. This doesn't mean they are rich, however, in anything other than land, fancy electronic milking equipment, cats, and cows. They are still cash-poor, as milk prices have been low for decades in Vermont.

I plop down next to his folding chair and say hi. Then I plunge in. "Do you ever think of switching to grass-fed beef and dairy?"

"Yeah, sometimes."

I tell him I pay $8 a pound for 100 percent grass-fed burger in the store, $5 directly to the farmers I buy from. Steaks are twice as much, or even more.

He whistles through his big brown beard. "I get less than two dollars a pound for mine!" he says, sounding like I might have piqued his interest. "But we are way too invested in our current setup to switch over."

"Yeah, I saw that article that you just got those new robotic milking machines. Sounds pretty wild."

He nods, "The machines keep us up at night—every time something goes wrong, an alarm goes off and I have to go check out who is stuck where. Sometimes I'm up every few hours."

"Of course!" I laugh. I can't say I'm surprised. Typical of modern life to save the farmer work during the day and lose him his sleep at night.

"What if you just used one portion of your land, as an experiment? You could even let some young farmer manage it."

"I couldn't afford to put cows on there," he says. "I need all my fields for growing corn for silage and hay for winter." He goes on to explain that pasture is at a premium these days. Big industrial farms are buying up all the land that he used to rent from other farmers.

A baseball flies over the fence and someone yells, "Heads up!"

Our goals overlap but are decidedly different. He is trying to stay afloat, economically, and keep his small dairy farm going in the face of large corporate interests so he can pass the family farm along to his children. This goal, if accomplished, would be a small miracle in this day and age. Farms the size of his have gone out of business at an alarming rate over the past few decades, with the beautiful rolling fields and barns sold off to real estate developers or larger agribusiness firms. The number of farms in Vermont has gone from 11,000 in the 1940s to fewer than 1,000 today.

In my mind, however, this conversation is part of my job as a health-care provider. Not only am I trying to lessen the economic stresses on his family, who are patients of mine; I'm also trying to improve the soil and water quality in our town, and create a more vibrant local food system for our whole community.

"Do any stores sell local grass-fed beef and dairy around here?" he asks. His question is telling—large silver trucks come to his farm daily, to pick up the milk and take it far away, paying him a pittance for it. Even though he and his partner are probably our largest local producers, he is completely out of the loop of the local food economy.

"Yes, lots of them do, even the gas station right here in town, and they sell out quickly. You probably wouldn't need more land, you might need even less."

"Hmm," he grunts, sounding doubtful.

"Ever heard of planned rotational grazing? You can put up to five times as many head of cattle on a piece of land, and it makes the fields more fertile for whatever else you decide to grow there in the future."

"Yeah, I've read articles about it."

I watch Alden pitch for half an inning. I know that Patrick is a quiet man, who only knows me through his wife and kids, and that this is a delicate subject, and an odd situation—a woman who grew up in an urban family trying to give advice to a farmer.

He breaks the silence. "On the fields where we do graze, we have started dividing them up a bit more and doing something a little bit like that. But not on the scale you are talking about."

Alden finally throws several strikes. He had a rough start.

"Did you see the article on the cover of *Time* magazine?" I ask.

"Nope."

"It's all about how beef and butter are okay to eat again, especially from grass-fed cows." The article explains that the theories about saturated fat causing heart disease were all wrong. I want Patrick to see that there really could be a market for this. "You know about the huge amounts of omega-3s in grass-fed beef?"

"Yes, from Kendra, she's all over that."

"Oh, of course."

Kendra, his wife, has been a friend and patient of mine for years. She came to me with endocrine-related fertility issues, and credits our acupuncture sessions and a nutrient-dense diet with helping her to finally get pregnant. We met twenty years ago when she was a bank teller across the street from my first office, down in the small business district of East Thetford, next door to what was then Gray's cattle auction. We were both starting out our careers. Since then she's been a waitress and the lunch lady at the elementary school; now she works extra hours at the pizza shop that the former police chief just opened.

Patrick and Kendra's son, Hunter, comes up to bat to start the seventh inning. He hits a ground ball through the infield for a single.

"You know, people always talk about 'grass-fed' animals . . . but corn *is* a grass," Patrick points out. "The grains are just much larger and more full of carbohydrates than other grasses."

"Yes, that's true," I say. I know this is a sore point in their family; that his kids are mad at their health teacher for assigning Michael Pollan articles to read, and for sharply criticizing farmers who feed cows corn. Given the tenseness around that issue, I decide not to criticize the corn itself. He is, in fact, correct. Corn, strange as it may seem, *is* a grass, an innocent grass that has been manipulated by corporations.

And corporations, ironically, are people.

"Only trouble with corn," I say, "is that farmers are dependent on some big corporation that sets the prices for it, when they could be independent. You could be making a living directly from the land you own, without needing to buy all those inputs."

Patrick nods. "That's true. There's only two companies that make everything now, and they can charge what they want. I pay $200 a bag for seeds."

"Can you save seeds from the corn you grow to plant the next year?" I know the answer to this, but some things are easier to let other people say. I don't want to criticize his ways, or even Monsanto's. I just want to offer another choice.

"Nope. The genetically engineered stuff is all patented. We don't harvest corn as a grain anyways, we harvest the whole plant and turn it into silage. We buy corn for grain by the tractor-trailer-full, and that has gone way up in price too."

"Why's that?"

"Ethanol."

"Oh yeah, ethanol. Not the brightest environmental idea ever to hit the planet."

It's his turn: "Yeah, it takes as much energy to grow the corn to produce ethanol as you get from it. Though I think if you made it from something else it might be more efficient. Corn is just so *easy*."

Three runs come in, and the other team, whose players all look bigger and stronger than our kids, is suddenly pulling way ahead of ours. The score is 20 to 6.

"You know about carbon farming, right?" It's pretty clear to me by now that Patrick doesn't need to be educated about any of this. If he's been reading about holistic grazing in his agricultural journals, I'm sure they have mentioned the ranchers, like Blain, who are using this practice specifically to move atmospheric carbon into the soil.

"Yup."

"Well last week both Congress and the State Department decided to look into it."

His bushy eyebrows shoot up and his eyes widen. Then narrow. He seems slightly suspicious, but he's clearly following the same rural social rules that I am.

"Is *that* right . . . " he says, in the Vermont way, which is more of a statement than a question.

"It's true! A friend of mine was at the meeting. I think the State Department is interested in it because it solves so many problems at once; food, water, desertification . . . it turns atmospheric CO_2 into living soil, and it helps prevent flooding and drought."

"Yeah, California is a mess. I'm glad we live in the Northeast, where we don't have to pay for irrigation."

"My guess is that if they really go for this as a major solution, there could be tax breaks for the farmers who are using it, but . . . the real reward is in the land productivity. From what I've seen, the soil will pay you even if the government doesn't."

"Something to think about," he says, stretching his arms and standing up as the game ends.

I agree. "Something to think about."

The teams are lining up, the panthers in their blue uniforms and the tigers in their gray ones, shaking each other's hands. We didn't win this game, but it's okay. The boys haven't lost their enthusiasm. It's only the beginning of the summer season.

Ecological Medicine Manifesto

Ecological medicine understands that we are part of a larger whole: a complex living system. This living system, like others, is self-organizing, intelligent, and constantly evolving.

Our bodies are a microsystem, reflective of—and nested within—the whole.

The health of any part of a system is intimately connected to the flows and processes of the whole. Therefore, to care for the environment is part of caring for ourselves and our patients.

Ecological medicine also recognizes that other self-organizing, intelligent communities live within us. Ecological medicine respects the right of all these communities—both inside and around us—to co-exist and collaborate.

Ecological medicine knows that connection is essential, and that disease is a manifestation of lack of connection. Each disconnection that occurs leads to a loss of power, integrity, flexibility, and energy—both for that part and for the whole. Therefore, to create health, one must restore connection.

Ecological medicine does this by:

- Acknowledging that networks, relationships, and communities exist at every level
- Facilitating communication, understanding, and cooperation within and between them
- Respecting the integrity and wisdom of community networks by using local knowledge and resources whenever possible

- Reconnecting people with the inherent wisdom and support of the social and natural communities that surround them

Health depends also on our ability to honor wildness, which has its own wisdom and integrity. Ecological medicine therefore seeks to restore the integrity, power, and sanctity of wild places—from the internal flora and fauna of the body, to the microorganisms of the soils, to the places and processes that plants, animals, and fungi depend on for survival, diversity, and well-being.

Ecological medicine respects and accepts that cycles of growth, decline, transformation, and regeneration are natural and essential to the health and balance of the entire system.

Ecological medicine operates best in environments that are fertile rather than sterile. It does this by encouraging honest, open-hearted, and evenly balanced relationships. And by recognizing that healthy communities are built through relationship, including cross-pollination of ideas, populations, and strategies for resilience.

Ecological medicine is regenerative, rather than extractive. Therefore, it focuses on processes rather than on products and profits.

Ecological medicine is affordable to learn, to practice, and to partake in, and care is available to all parts of the system.

Ecological medicine is flexible and adaptive, and therefore is interested in, and responsive to, individual and local circumstances.

When disease occurs, ecological medicine looks for patterns, not individually occurring symptoms. To do this, ecological medicine gathers information from the whole system. When looking at a single part, ecological medicine understands that within each part, the whole is reflected, as well.

Ecological medicine works within the patterns of nature, not against them, and does not exploit one part of the system for the purposes of another.

Ecological medicine is slow medicine. It begins with deep listening and understanding, and it allows time for deep and lasting cures.

ACKNOWLEDGMENTS

A few people have put in more than their fair share of time and love on this book:

Karen Thorkilsen donated many hours as an editor in the very early and very late stages of the book, and took me seriously in a way that has stayed with me.

Donlon Wade encouraged me to write a book, cheered me on, and helped me learn to enjoy solitude enough to get it done.

Katie Williams drove me to and from my early talks on the subject, listened to me as I tried to gather my ideas at the last minute, and coached me on how to say things more succinctly.

Scott Graham coached me for many unpaid hours early in the project in setting up a writer's schedule.

Mark Kutolowski offered his editorial support, as well as his couch, laundry facilities, woodstove, and quiet house to write in, book-related loans, brisk walks, long talks, prayers, and cold swims.

Kerstin Lipke put in many hours of editing and a huge amount of emotional and logistical support.

Julé Anne Creem mopped up buckets of tears and kept me hopeful. I have no idea what I would have done without her.

George Dimock propped me up against mountains of internalized sexism, and wisely counseled me out of my fears of academic critics looking down their nose at me and my worries about other people stealing my ideas.

My mother, Lisa Dittrich, read drafts, encouraged me, and inspired me with her own creativity and brave social change work. She is an all-around amazing mother.

My stepfather, Olda Dittrich, stepped in at crucial times, urged me on, kept me on task, bailed me out of my messes, coached me as I developed ideas about health care and economics, and never gave up even though I crashed past every deadline he tried to set for me.

My sons, Henry and Alden Nichols, listened, brainstormed,

edited, proofread, cheered my successes, wrote and finished many of their own projects, and never said a discouraging word to me even though they spent more than half of their childhoods waiting for me to finish this project. (When I did finish, I said, "I feel like I have had an owl sitting on my head for most of your childhood," to which Alden replied simply: "That's a good analogy.")

Marisa Hebb helped me understand and connect to a new generation of leaders, created my fund-raising video, edited an early draft, worked on footnotes, and kept the mundane details of my life moving forward.

Lynda Day Martin listened to chapters, commented, thought together with me, did a lot of research, and kept me laughing as we walked up hills together. She was the reader I had in mind as I wrote this.

Bob Stein alternately cheered me on, left me alone, and fed me during the final stages of the first draft, while challenging me to go "deeper into the dark heart of the material." When I asked him if he thought it would ever be done, he said, "No." Then he paused, looking at my crestfallen face, and added, "But at some point you *will* decide to stop. And then you will write the book you *really* want to write." (We'll see . . .)

Laure Stevens-Lubin, Dale Gephart, Telisa Stewart, Dan Bednarz, Lisa Frost, Adam Lake, Carol Egbert, and Cynthia Keith read, commented on, and copyedited chapters and drafts.

Makenna Goodman, Brianne Goodspeed, Joni Praded, and Margo Baldwin at Chelsea Green were foster parents to the first draft of this book.

Mark Morgan at SuperTechX fixed many computers over and over again, always in a timely fashion. His technical support was worth much more than he charged me.

Eric Rickstad restored my writer's ego at a crucial moment, and tried to untangle an enormous first draft.

Joni Cole did the impossible and pulled it all together into an actual structure.

Jeri Helen did a beautiful job of copyediting.

Ruby Levesque at Random House spent many, many hours designing a beautiful cover.

Peter Holm at Sterling Hill opened up his schedule and then patiently waited for the manuscript, several times over.

Lucy Gardner Carson was the best, most nitpicking copy-editor and proofreader anyone could ever hope for [and she never held it against me if I chose to ignore her suggestions—lgc].

Peter Donovan provided wonderful drawings, upped the ante in my scientific quests, and opened my life to include heart-warming journeys in the beloved bus and beyond.

I am indebted to all the patients who have supported my practice for twenty-two years and taught me most everything I know about how people heal.

I am grateful also for Nick Delbanco and all the writers and artists at Vermont Studio Center, as well as Cora Brooks, Allan Hoving, Jim Schley, Joe Elliot, Duncan Nichols, Will Allen, Judy Schwartz, Kristen Ohlsen, Janisse Ray, Pat Freund, and many other fellow writers, for encouraging me. I especially appreciate Amelia Bullmore, who matched my prolific transatlantic letter-writing tendencies from when we were nine years old until the Internet was invented.

For my father, Derek, who taught me to notice and love the little details of life (like the smell of one's own knees in a bathtub). For my fabulous siblings, Ben, Edward, Laska, Luke, and Sarah, who inspire me and keep my sense of humor intact, for my stepmother Gayle who taught me many skills, for my alternate parents Pamela and Jeremy Bullmore and Scott and Betsy Harshbarger, and all the amazing great-aunts and grand-women who helped raise me.

For the friends and family who were looking forward to reading this book, but whom I lost while I was still writing it: Emily Scoville, Grace Paley, Bob Nichols (who, even on his deathbed, kept telling me I needed an editor), Don Dickey (who introduced me to the concept of a "community of practice" which is really the heart and soul of this book), Tipi Halsey, David Rakoff (the first real fan of my writing, who used to leave me love notes on my door in college after my poetry readings), Alex Dickey, Eva Behrens, Leonard Hanitchak, John Joline, Pat Freund, Nina Swaim, and Winnie Aaronian. I wish I had finished it sooner.

For my many other current and past daily/weekly/monthly supporters, friends, and co-listeners, including Belinda Ray, Claudia Henrion, Sarah Ireland, Vanessa Rule, Mary Beth Hassett, Alison Baker, Paula O'Brien, Rebecca Lovejoy, Meghan Wilson, Anna Goldstein, Seth Itzkan, Leo Daly, Abigail Feldman, Theresa Krieger, Claudia Marieb, Sean Dalton, Kerstin Nichols, Kathy Manns, the health-care workers at the Good Neighbor Clinic and White River Family Practice, Ruth Gibbud, Justin Evans, Niko Horster, Bill Keegan, Liana Horster, Barb Delzio, Pam Parker, Doris Anderson, Amelia Sereen, Marilyn McEnery, Joanie Hebb, Goizalde Galartza, Amanda Calder, Nancy Gabriel, Deb Robinson, Jay Cary, Jen Hauck, Lorraine Carbino, Michelle Billings, Nora Kovacs, Mary Mathieu, Sue Wolfe, Myron Moore, Julia Duran Arellano, Jill Brose, Gina DiMaria, Cristia Lesher, David Stringham, Deana Rich, Mahala Mazerov, Carol Jackson, Maureen Burford, Charlie Shepard, Robert Hayden, Spero Latchis, Chris Hollis, Julie Forbes, Marisa Sullivan, Michael Jackman, Eliza Gagnon, Checker Ives, Nika Annon, Debi Hoffman, Jim Vanderpool, Karen Caplan, Tiki Fuhro, Winnie Aaronian, and many others.

For all my teachers, mentors, and inspiring colleagues, including (but by no means limited to) Maurice Page, Peggy Umanzio, Ted Martin, Larry Aaronson, Lorraine Ballard, Dinah Vaprin, Sidney Mackenzie, Robbee Fian, Brewster Beach, Barbara Stoler Miller, Jayesh Shah, Koei Kuwahara, Takahashi Sensei, Swami Asokananda, Dan Nickerson, Sister Elizabeth Oleksak, David Jernigan, Suzanne Serat, Lu Wei Dong, Shou Chun Ma, Sharon Weizenbaum, Andy Gamble, Glenn Rothfeld, Russ Vernon-Jones, Joanna Waldman, Joette Hayashigawa, Beth Edmunds, Mary Hodgson, Elaine Ingham, Diane Balser, Diane Shisk, John Sellen, Jo Saunders, Christine Jones, Allan Savory, Walter Jehne, Ray

Archuleta, Gwen Brown, Teresa Enrico, Foster Brown, Adam Lake, Jonathan Lundgren, Precious Phiri, Blaine and Naomi Hjertaas, Neil Dennis, Trent and Carolyn Wall, Ralph and Lynda Corcoran, George Whitten, Julie Sullivan, Trudi and John Kretsinger, Joe and Julie Morris, Gabe Brown, and Gail Fuller.

I am especially appreciative of the many, many innovative health-care workers, farmers, ranchers, teachers, and other hard-working people I have met who are doing the hands-on work of regenerating the world. (I will be writing about you all in much more detail in the future.)

Huge thanks to the following people who contributed financially to this project through crowd-source funding and personal donations. Some of you I've known for years, some of you I've never met. All of you brought tears to my eyes.

Cheryl Hill Nation, Peter Parise, Cynthia Greer, Abigail Feldman, Barb and Jerry Vidal, Andy Rowles, Brenda Loew, Biggie Arnold, Carey Harben, Diana Di Gioia, Chris Hollis, Hao Xu, Helen Quigley, Howard Chesshire, Jane Morgan, Jeanette W. Moy, Joan Ashley, Joanna Rueter, Julie and Ella Forbes, Larry Forbes, Kerstin Nichols, Liana Hebb, Lisa Dittrich, Lucy Vaughters, Marilyn Cook, Martin Feldman, Nancy Gabriel, Mark Kutolowski, Christine Esten, Olda Dittrich, Ray Chin, Ridge Satterthwaite, Mary Wunderlich, Sharon Weizenbaum, Shirley Gramling, Suzanne Kates, Tracy Brown, Marie Ptackova, Nicky Corrao, Sylvia Davatz, Gary Huang-Dale, Anna Goldstein, Anne Mulkerrin, Bela Toth, Bob Stein, Bria Gabriel Singer, Cynthia Keith, Christine Cowles, Dale Gephart, Debra L. Diegoli, Heidi Luquer, Jennifer Dembinski, Joy and Ted Gaine, Julia Greenspan, Julie Kienitz, Kathy Blume, Mark Krawczyk, Mary Beth Hassett, Mary Lee Vigent, Mary Ruggles, Nick Robson, Nicole Andrade, Nora Jacobson, Patricia Seykora, Perry Allison, Phil Haskins, Rebecca Lovejoy, Sally Duston and Dean Whitlock, Sarah Pershouse, Derek Pershouse, Sheena Chaffee, Stephanie Carney, Steven Jackman, Susan Breslow, Sylvia Davatz, Teresa Quintanilla, Tracy Thorne,

Zed Zabski, Robert Hayden, Spero Latchis, Karen Van Houten, Gillian Tyler, Phillip Glaser, Susan Davidson, Robert Hayden, Chris Esten and Boots Wardinski, Swami Asokananda, Richard Michalski, "In memory of Marsha Lee," Eliza Gagnon, Alexander Dickey, Felice Silverman, Terry Osborne, Bruce Harrow, Douglas Lovell, Sylvia Davatz, "In memory of Connor Cook," Bob Bauer, Catherine Shields, John Rogers, Mahala Mazerov, Cheryl Conner, David Rossi, Jane Applegate, Keith and Sherry Merrick, Nina Swaim and Doug Smith, Freddie and Arthur Steinberg, Jody Biddle, Kye Cochran, Ursula Rudd, Deb Meyer, Jools Skeet, Robert Ferris, Mark and Amy McElroy, Bob Watson, and many others who chose to remain anonymous.

Finally, I am grateful for Phoebe, the dog who kept me warm and waited patiently for so many walks.

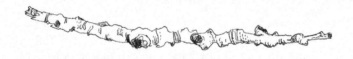

ABOUT THE AUTHOR

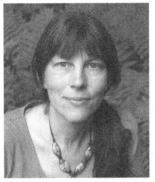 Didi Pershouse is the founder of the Center for Sustainable Medicine, where she developed a model for systems-based ecological medicine that restores health to individuals as well as the social and natural communities around them. Over the past 22 years, her health-care practice has expanded in its scope from treating individual patients to treating whole systems.

In addition to raising two sons and seeing patients in Thetford Center, Vermont, she also travels and teaches around the continent with the Soil Carbon Coalition. She teaches about the interrelationships between healthy soils, shifting weather patterns, economic forces, and human health; trains community leaders in self-care and peer support; develops curricula about biological work and landscape function; and works with farmers and ranchers to restore the living systems that run the underground carbon and water cycles that make life on this planet possible.

ABOUT THE ILLUSTRATOR

Peter Donovan is the founder of the Soil Carbon Coalition. He has herded sheep, played piano for ballet classes, and worked on cattle ranches, but he now spends most of his time touring North America in his school-bus home, facilitating workshops, and measuring changes in soil carbon and water cycles. The drawings in this book are from his travels. He has reported widely on innovative land managers; most of his articles can be found at managingwholes.com.

Made in the USA
Las Vegas, NV
10 April 2024

88495127R00184